Transforming Health Markets in Asia and Africa

There has been a dramatic spread of health markets in much of Asia and Africa over the past couple of decades. This has substantially increased the availability of health-related goods and services in all but the most remote localities, but it has created problems with safety, efficiency and cost. The effort to bring order to these chaotic markets is almost certain to become one of the greatest challenges in global health.

This book documents the problems associated with unregulated health markets and presents innovative approaches that have emerged to address them. It outlines a framework that researchers, policy-makers and social entrepreneurs can use to analyse health market systems and assess the likely outcome of alternative interventions. The book presents a new way of understanding highly marketized health systems, applies this understanding to an analysis of health markets in countries across Asia and Africa, and identifies some of the major new developments for making these markets perform better in meeting the needs of the poor. It argues that it is time to move beyond ideological debates about the roles of public and private sectors in an ideal health system and focus more on understanding the operation of these markets and developing practical strategies for improving their performance.

This book is ideal reading for researchers and students in public health, development studies, public policy and administration, health economics, medical anthropology, and science and technology studies. It is also a valuable resource for policy-makers, social entrepreneurs, and planners and managers in public- and private-sector health systems, including pharmaceutical companies, aid agencies, NGOs and international organizations.

Gerald Bloom is a Fellow of the Institute of Development Studies. He leads the IDS team in the Future Health Systems Consortium and convenes the health domain of the STEPS Centre at the University of Sussex.

Barun Kanjilal is Professor of Health Economics at the Indian Institute for Health Management Research in Jaipur.

Henry Lucas is a Researcher at the Institute of Development Studies in the Future Health Systems Consortium, focusing on social protection and health, and the application of new technologies.

David H. Peters is Director of the Health Systems Programme in the Department of International Health of the Johns Hopkins School of Public Health and Director of the Future Health Systems Consortium.

Pathways to Sustainability Series

This book series addresses core challenges around linking science and technology and environmental sustainability with poverty reduction and social justice. It is based on the work of the Social, Technological and Environmental Pathways to Sustainability (STEPS) Centre, a major investment of the UK Economic and Social Research Council (ESRC). The STEPS Centre brings together researchers at the Institute of Development Studies (IDS) and SPRU (Science and Technology Policy Research) at the University of Sussex with a set of partner institutions in Africa, Asia and Latin America.

Series Editors:
Melissa Leach, Ian Scoones and Andy Stirling
STEPS Centre at the University of Sussex

Editorial Advisory Board:
Steve Bass, Wiebe E. Bijker, Victor Galaz, Wenzel Geissler,
Katherine Homewood, Sheila Jasanoff, Colin McInnes, Suman Sahai,
Andrew Scott

Titles in this series include:

Dynamic Sustainabilities
Technology, environment, social justice
Melissa Leach, Ian Scoones and Andy Stirling

Avian Influenza
Science, policy and politics
Edited by Ian Scoones

Rice Biofortification
Lessons for global science and development
Sally Brooks

Epidemics
Science, governance and social justice
Edited by Sarah Dry and Melissa Leach

Contested Agronomy
Agricultural research in a changing world
James Sumberg and John Thompson

Transforming Health Markets in Asia and Africa
Improving quality and access for the poor
Edited by Gerald Bloom, Barun Kanjilal, Henry Lucas and David H. Peters

Pastoralism and Development in Africa
Dynamic change at the margins
Edited by Ian Scoones, Andy Catley and Jeremy Lind

Transforming Health Markets in Asia and Africa

Improving quality and access for the poor

Edited by Gerald Bloom,
Barun Kanjilal, Henry Lucas
and David H. Peters

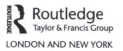

LONDON AND NEW YORK

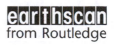

First edition published 2013
by Routledge
2 Park Square, Milton Park, Abingdon, Oxon, OX14 4RN

Simultaneously published in the USA and Canada
by Routledge
711 Third Avenue, New York, NY 10017

Routledge is an imprint of the Taylor & Francis Group, an informa business

British Library Cataloguing in Publication Data
A catalogue record for this book is available from the British Library

Library of Congress Cataloging-in-Publication Data
Transforming health markets in Asia and Africa : improving quality and
access for the poor / Gerald Bloom ... [et al.]. – 1st ed.
p. ; cm.
Includes bibliographical references.
I. Bloom, Gerald .
[DNLM: 1. Health Care Sector–Africa. 2. Health Care Sector–Asia.
3. Health Services Needs and Demand–Africa. 4. Health Services Needs
and Demand–Asia. 5. Developing Countries--Africa. 6. Developing
Countries–Asia. 7. Health Care Reform--Africa. 8. Health Care Reform–Asia.
9. Health Services Accessibility--Africa. 10. Health Services
Accessibility–Asia. W 84 JA1]
362.1'042–dc23
2012006705

ISBN13: 978–1–84971–416–7 (hbk)
ISBN13: 978–1–84971–417–4 (pbk)
ISBN13: 978–0–203–10206–0 (ebk)

Typeset in Times New Roman by
Keystroke, Station Road, Codsall, Wolverhampton

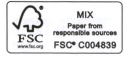

Printed and bound in Great Britain by the MPG Books Group

Contents

Illustrations

Figures

Tables

Boxes

Contributors

Smisha Agarwal is a Carl E. Taylor Memorial Fellow working at the Comprehensive Rural Health Project (CRHP), Jamkhed, India, developing effective monitoring and evaluation systems for community-based programmes. She is co-founder of Global Health Bridge, a non-profit organization focused on using technology to improve health services delivery.

Owasim Akram is currently working as Research Coordinator for Plan International. He received the award of best research poster at the Eighth International Urban Health Conference, Nairobi, October 2009, which focused on men's sexual health in Bangladesh.

Rumesa Rowen Aziz has a BA in Liberal Arts from Hampshire College and an MFA from Hunter College of the City University of New York. She has five years of professional experience in public health research with a focus on health equity and community empowerment.

Abbas Bhuiya is a Senior Social Scientist. He is the Head of the Poverty and Health Programme and Social and Behavioural Sciences Unit, as well as the Deputy Executive Director, of ICDDR,B.

David M. Bishai is a Professor in the Department of Population and Family and Reproductive Health at the Johns Hopkins University Bloomberg School of Public Health. He is a member of the American Economics Association, the International Health Economics Association and the American Public Health Association. He is a Fellow of the American Academy of Pediatrics and a Fellow of the American College of Physicians, and he continues a part-time clinical practice in Towson, MD.

Gerald Bloom, a medical doctor and health systems analyst, is a Fellow of the Institute of Development Studies in Brighton, UK. He has worked for many years on the health style reform and development in complex and rapidly changing contexts. He leads the IDS team in the Future Health Systems Consortium and convenes the health domain of the STEPS Centre at the University of Sussex.

Claire Champion has over twelve years of experience designing and implementing technical and organizational strategies for health systems strengthening in the public and private sectors and facilitating cross-sectoral partnerships. She has a Master of Business Administration from Harvard Business School and a Doctorate of Public Health from Johns Hopkins University.

Fang Jing earned her PhD at the Institute of Development Studies (IDS), the University of Sussex, UK, in 2006. She has undertaken research on Chinese rural healthcare services, particularly women's reproductive health services, for two decades, and has provided technical support for projects undertaken by the Chinese National Family Planning Commission and Ministry of Health, as well as several international organizations. She is also a WHO adviser for the Gender and Rights Advisory Panel and member of the executive editorial group of the journal *EcoHealth*.

Fang Lijie, who has a PhD in Sociology, is a Researcher at the Institute of Sociology in the Chinese Academy of Social Sciences, Beijing. Her research focused on health systems and health policy for a number of years. Her current work concerns the transition of the entire social welfare system.

Sayed Manzoor Ahmed Hanifi is an Assistant Scientist currently working in the Centre for Equity and Health System at ICDDR,B. He is a Coordinator of the research group Methods and Measurements.

Mohammad Iqbal has been working as Deputy Project Coordinator at the Centre for Equity and Health Systems at ICDDR,B. He is also serving as a coordinator of the Universal Health Coverage Research Group at the same centre. He has nearly twenty-five years of experience in public health and research, with special focus on health systems and health equity.

Barun Kanjilal works at the Indian Institute of Health Management Research (IIHMR), Jaipur, India, as Professor of Health Economics and Health Systems Research. He obtained his PhD (Economics) from Louisiana State University, USA. He is currently working as Coordinator of the Future Health Systems (FHS) Research Project Consortium in India.

Henry Lucas, a statistician who specializes in information systems, monitoring and evaluation, and research methods, is a Fellow of the Institute of Development Studies in Brighton, UK. His work has focused on health and health systems for many years and he is an active participant in the Future Health Systems Consortium.

Shehrin Shaila Mahmood is an Assistant Scientist of ICDDR,B and is currently a PhD candidate at the Australian National University. As a social science researcher she has over ten years of experience in the field of health and development research. She has published several articles in peer-reviewed journals on topics related to poverty and health, health equity, health systems and healthcare provision.

Sumit Mazumdar is currently a Fellow at the Institute for Human Development, New Delhi. Earlier, he taught courses on Indian economic development at the

Indian Institute of Technology, Mandi. He has worked as Consultant with the Future Health Systems Research Project Consortium, IIHMR-Kolkata, and the Centre for Studies in Social Sciences, Calcutta.

Chean Men is a PhD candidate trained in the field of medical anthropology, specializing in qualitative research. He is one of the founding members of MoPoTsyo, a Cambodian NGO that supports people with diabetes in rural communities. He is also involved in an ongoing evaluation of MoPoTsyo's peer education intervention on chronic diseases.

Oladimeji Oladepo is Professor of Public Health, and Dean of the Faculty of Public Health, University of Ibadan, Nigeria. He is the FHS Consortium focal point for malaria and patent medicine vendor (PMV) informal health market research. In the past few years he has conducted qualitative and quantitative studies on innovative interventions and policy modification on patent medicine vendors' informal markets in Nigeria, working closely with governments and international agencies.

David H. Peters is currently Director and Associate Chair of the Health Systems Program, and Professor of International Health in the Department of International Health, Johns Hopkins University, Bloomberg School of Public Health, Baltimore. He is also Adjunct Professor at the International Institute of Health Management and Research, Delhi.

M. Hafizur Rahman, faculty member at the Johns Hopkins University, is a public health physician with more than fifteen years of experience in directing health systems research and programs in low- and middle-income countries. As a faculty member of Johns Hopkins School of Medicine, he has been involved in clinical research with the colleagues from Johns Hopkins School of Medicine.

Zeeshan Rahman has an MA in Political Science from York University, Canada. In recent years he has been involved with human development research work focusing on governance and human rights, social development, and global health issues.

Sabina Faiz Rashid, Professor at the James P. Grant School of Public Health, BRAC University, has been working in Bangladesh since 1993. Since 2007 she has been teaching a course at the Berlin School of Public Health at Charité, Germany. In 2011 she became an Adjunct Visiting Faculty, Professorial Lecturer in Global Health at George Washington University, Washington, DC.

Ren Jing received her Master's degree from the China Medical University in 2006, majoring in Social Medicine and Health Management. Since then she has been working for the Ministry of Health, carrying out research on rural health and the New Rural Cooperative Medical Scheme (NRCMS), a rural social health insurance in China covering a rural population of 830 million.

Mohammad Sohel Shomik has been working as Research Investigator at the Centre for Child and Adolescent Health at ICDDR,B. He is also a Field

Manager of Mirzapur Filed Site at the same centre. He has nearly eight years of experience in public health and research with special focus on health system management.

Hilary Standing is a social scientist and social anthropologist. She has worked extensively in India and Bangladesh. She specializes in health and development and has worked on health systems issues in several countries. She is a researcher on the Johns Hopkins University-led DFID Research Programme Consortium on Future Health Systems. Until 2010 she was a professorial fellow at the Institute of Development Studies, University of Sussex. She is now a visiting Fellow and Emeritus Professor.

Wim Van Damme is a Professor in Public Health, teaching health policy at the Institute of Tropical Medicine, Antwerp, Belgium. He has worked for ten years overseas with Médecins sans Frontières in Peru, Sudan, Guinea and Cambodia.

Maurits van Pelt is one of the founding members of the Cambodian non-governmental organization MoPoTsyo Patient Information Centre and has been its Executive Director since its inception. He holds a Master's degree in law from Vrije Universiteit in Amsterdam and one in health policy planning and financing from the London School of Hygiene and Tropical Medicine and London School of Economics.

Tania Wahed is currently studying for a PhD in the United States. She worked as Senior Operations Researcher at the Social and Behavioural Sciences Unit at ICDDR,B between August 2008 and March 2011. She has nearly fifteen years of experience in teaching and research with special focus on health equity and economic consequences of health care.

Ou Vun is currently Provincial Health Adviser with the Deutsche Gesellschaft für Internationale Zusammenarbeit's (GIZ) Social Health Protection Program in Kampot Province in Cambodia. He has a long-standing and very broad experience in the development of Cambodia's health sector that spans almost thirty years. He obtained his doctoral degree in 1988 and trained in Thailand, Japan and Belgium.

Wu Huazhang is Professor and Head of Teaching at the Research Section of Health Care Management of China Medical University (CMU). He is a board member of the Academic Committee of the China Health Economics Association, a member of the expert panel of the China Health Economics Training and Research Network, and an editorial member of the *Journal of China Health Economics* and two other national academic journals. He has received the award of Liaoning Province Youth Talent on Philosophy and Social Science.

Acknowledgements

This book is an output of the Future Health Systems Research Programme Consortium and the STEPS Centre. It has benefited greatly from a number of discussions over several years between the authors of the chapters and other researchers from the Future Health Systems Research Programme Consortium. We have also benefited from our association with the STEPS Centre, which has offered continuous intellectual stimulation. Several of the authors presented their ideas to a conference entitled Beyond Scaling Up in Brighton in May 2010, hosted jointly by the Future Health Systems Consortium and the STEPS Centre, and they benefited greatly from excellent comments from conference participants. We also presented some of the findings to the First Global Symposium on Health Systems Research in November 2010 and benefited from the many comments we received.

The production of the book would not have been possible without the unfailing support of Jan Boyes. She maintained communications with authors living on three continents and played a key role in editing and formatting the entire book. The authors of several chapters owe a debt of gratitude to Tendayi Bloom, who helped them rewrite their papers to make them more accessible.

We would like to acknowledge two sources of funding that have made the production of this book possible. The STEPS Centre, with support from the Economic and Social Research Council in the United Kingdom, provided financial support for the conference Beyond Scaling Up, which played a key role in the development of several of the chapters. It has also supported the publication of the book as part of a series. Funding provided by the Department of International Development in the United Kingdom for the Future Health Systems Research Programme Consortium enabled partners to undertake studies in India, Bangladesh and Nigeria, and also supported the authors in writing this book. The contents of the book are the sole responsibility of the authors and the editors.

Abbreviations

ACT	artemisinin-combined therapy
AEH	Aravind Eye Hospitals
AIDS	acquired immunodeficiency syndrome
ARV	antiretroviral
BBS	Bangladesh Bureau of Statistics
BBUASM	Bangladesh Board of Unani and Ayurvedic Systems of Medicine
BMDC	Bangladesh Medical and Dental Council
BNC	Bangladesh Nursing Council
BP	blood pressure
BPC	Bangladesh Pharmacy Council
BPL	below the poverty line
CAGR	compound annual growth rate
CT	computerized tomography
DD	drug detailer
DFID	Department for International Development (United Kingdom)
DIC	Disciplinary Inspection Committee
DPM	diabetes programme manager
EHR	electronic health record
EMR	electronic medical record
FBG	fasting blood glucose
FDI	foreign direct investment
FDRA	Food and Drug Regulatory Agency
FGD	focus-group discussion
FHS	Future Health Systems
FMOH	Federal Ministry of Health
FWV	family welfare visitor
GDP	gross domestic product
GI	glycaemic index
GMP	Good Manufacturing Practice
GSMF	Ghana Social Marketing Foundation
GTZ	Deutsche Gesellschaft für Technische Zusammenarbeit
HDSS	Health and Demographic Surveillance System
HI	health inspector

HIV	human immunodeficiency virus
ICDDR,B	International Centre for Diarrhoeal Disease Research, Bangladesh
ICT	information and communication technology
IDI	in-depth interview
IIHMR	Indian Institute of Health Management Research
IMCI	integrated management of childhood illness
IMR	infant mortality rate
IUD	intrauterine device
KFW	Kreditanstalt für Wiederaufbau
KMET	Kisumu Medical Education Trust
LMICs	low- and middle-income countries
LTFQ	less than fully qualified
MBBS	Bachelor of Medicine, Bachelor of Surgery
MD	Medical Doctor
MDG	Millennium Development Goal
MMR	maternal mortality ratio
MR	medical representative; menstrual regulation
MSF	Médicins sans Frontières
NCMS	New Cooperative Medical System
NFHS	National Family Health Survey
NGO	Non-Governmental Organization
NMCP	National Malaria Control Program
NRCMS	New Rural Cooperative Medical Scheme
NSAID	non-steroidal anti-inflammatory drug
NSSO	National Sample Survey Organisation (India)
OECD	Organisation for Economic Co-operation and Development
OOPS	out-of-pocket (health) spending
PBG	postprandial blood glucose
PDA	personal data assistant
PHARIA	Pharmaceutical Representative Association
PHC	primary health care
PMC	pharmaceutical multinational corporation
PMV	patent medicine vendor
POVILL	Poverty and Illness
PPP	public–private partnership
PSI	Population Services International
R&D	research and development
RIPEO	Rectifying Incorrect Professional Ethics Office
RMP	rural medical practitioner
Rs	rupees
RSBY	Rashtriya Swasthya Bima Yojana
RTBI	Rural Technology and Business Incubator
SACMO	sub-assistant community medical officer
SEZ	Special Economic Zone

SMF	State Medical Faculty
SMP	Social Marketing Pakistan
SMS	Short Message Service
SRH	sexual and reproductive health
SS	*ShasthyaSena*
SSC	Secondary School Certificate
STD	sexually transmitted disease
STI	sexually transmitted infection
THC	Thana Health Complex
TPA	third-party administrator
TRIPS	Trade-Related Aspects of Intellectual Property Rights
UC	union committee
UCLA	University of California, Los Angeles
UN	United Nations
USAID	US Agency for International Development
VD	village doctor
WHO	World Health Organization
WRI	World Resources Institute

1   Introduction

Gerald Bloom, Barun Kanjilal,
Henry Lucas, David H. Peters
and Hilary Standing

Introduction

This book is an output of the collaboration between the Future Health Systems Consortium and the STEPS Centre in a series of studies of the rapidly emerging health markets in Africa and Asia and the management of health system change in dynamic and complex contexts. The work arose out of consultations with national advisory groups in several countries and several workshops for researchers and policy-makers, which identified a lack of systematic evidence on the performance of these markets in meeting the health needs of the poor. The studies focus particularly on the very large informal markets through which the poor obtain a large proportion of their medical care. This book has been organized to provide a combination of case studies and overviews of certain aspects of the dynamic reality of health markets.

During the past two decades there has been a dramatic spread of market relationships in the health sector of many low- and middle-income countries (Mackintosh and Koivusalo, 2005). Typically, out-of-pocket payments account for a large proportion of total health expenditure, and a big share of healthcare transactions include some form of cash payment (National Health Accounts, 2007). Many countries have pluralistic health systems in which providers of health-related goods and services vary widely in terms of their practice settings, their type of knowledge and associated training, and their relationship with the legal system (Bloom and Standing, 2001). The spread of health-related markets has created both opportunities and challenges for improving the performance of health systems in relation to poor people. It has produced easier access to drugs and some form of medical advice for those who can pay. There are examples of excellent market-driven services, but, as Das *et al.* (2008) document, the quality of services both public and private health workers provide is often poor: the services are ineffective or dangerous.

The policies of some international organizations in supporting strict limits to government expenditure and advocating an increased role for health-related markets have arguably influenced these developments. But this phenomenon is widely associated with the rapid spread of market relationships in many countries. In some cases its emergence has been linked to the failure of state-provided health services to meet popular expectations. In other cases it is associated with a rapid spread of markets with economic growth. The spread of markets has often been much faster than the capacity of the state and other key actors to establish regulatory arrangements to influence their performance. A large proportion of market transactions now take place outside any national legal regulatory framework or in settings where regulatory regimes are poorly implemented or lack clarity. A common feature is also the blurring of boundaries between public and private sectors, with staff moving across these boundaries, often informally and sometimes in the course of one day, and users making informal payments for services or drugs at public facilities, or consulting government health workers 'privately'.

Much analysis of healthcare markets draws heavily on the experiences of the advanced market economies where there is a clearer demarcation of the roles of, and boundaries between, the public and private sectors in delivering services. This has led to a tendency to seek models for 'working with the private sector' from these countries, without taking sufficient account of their strong institutional and regulatory arrangements for both market and non-market services (Bloom and Standing, 2008).

This book takes a different approach, basing the assessment of the likely outcome of different reform options on a closer understanding of the realities of the markets that have emerged in developing and transitional economies. It focuses particularly on their performance in meeting the needs of the poor. It has two main aims. The first is to develop an exploratory framework for understanding how health markets operate in these contexts, primarily using a political economy rather than a public health approach to health systems. The argument rests on our view that theoretical perspectives grounded in an understanding of the dynamics of markets and their interplay with different contextual conditions offer fresh insights for health systems development. The second is to begin to lay out the implications of these different ways of thinking about health markets for policies and programmes. This points us away from standard health policy approaches to planning and regulation and towards questions of knowledge transfer and learning in highly dynamic environments.

Markets, institutions and health systems

This section provides a brief background to past and current debates about how health markets function. In particular, we note – and raise some problems with – the dominance of thinking drawn from the experience of the advanced market economies with long histories of regulation.

The limits of markets

The advanced market economies have created complex institutional arrangements within which state, market and civil society actors cooperate to translate scientific medical knowledge into widely accessible goods and expert services (Bloom *et al.*, 2008). Debates about health system organization, based on a combination of economic theory and historical evidence, have led to a widely held consensus on why markets, in themselves, do not produce efficient or equitable health systems.

The health sector is characterized by a number of well-understood 'market failures' (Bennett *et al.*, 1997). Government functions and other formal arrangements have arisen to compensate for these failures. For example, a variety of non-market institutions have developed to prevent possessors of expert knowledge from abusing their power, including professional self-regulation and internalized codes of ethics, public provision of services, government regulation and tort law. These institutions and mechanisms are also present, to some degree, in many low- and middle-income countries. In addition, markets have capacity for self-regulation on the basis that market share is often protected by demonstrated adherence to rules and standards. Again, institutions for creating greater market order are present in low- and middle-income countries, but in many contexts they are largely informal and predominantly local. Health system analysts have paid much less attention to the operation of informal health markets.

Box 1.1 'Market failures' in the health sector

- Health-related services include public goods, such as public sewerage and water supply systems, that would be undersupplied if left to the market.
- Services such as immunization have positive externalities in that an individual's consumption confers benefits on others, so that decisions based only on individual needs are likely to result in sub-optimal funding.
- Markets tend to under-insure against major health expenditure because they cannot control costs effectively and there is little incentive for a healthy person to join an insurance scheme.
- Markets may not adequately reflect the greater willingness of the population to finance basic health care than other, non-health goods and services.
- Markets can worsen distributive outcomes and hence health inequities.
- Markets for goods and services that embody expert knowledge produce information asymmetry between providers and clients that can make clients vulnerable to abuse of provider power.

'Path dependency' and institutional change

The experience of the advanced market economies provides useful insights into the problems of health systems in low- and middle-income countries, but it is dangerous to assume that the development of their institutions will follow a similar path. The concept of path dependency of technology (David, 1985) and institutions (Pierson and Skocpol, 2002; Thelen, 2003) describes the process by which a small early decision profoundly influences future development because of the increasing returns to institutionalization and the high cost of changing to a different path. The dominant model of health system organization is an example of path dependency: highly regulated professions and pharmaceutical markets reflect the social and economic context and associated institutional decisions within which the first modern health systems were embedded. It is important to keep this in mind when attempting to adapt institutional arrangements from one context to another and when assessing the likely future consequences of reforms.

Institutional arrangements in the health sector are notoriously 'sticky', mainly because they reflect the intrinsically political nature of health system reforms. Substantial resistance to change by stakeholder groups must be expected, where reforms might threaten their existence and the ideological stances that have evolved to justify the existing organizational arrangements (Altenstetter and Busse, 2005; Gordon, 2005; Rochaix and Wilsford, 2005). During the second half of the twentieth century, the right to health care became a highly charged political issue and governments became heavily involved in health financing and service delivery. The high political profile of health may have slowed the rate of institutional change. This could explain why health systems in advanced market economies preserve many aspects of their early-twentieth-century structure, while the organization of other economic and social sectors has changed much more.

The tendency of health systems to be path dependent has important implications for policy analysts in low- and middle-income countries. First, *frameworks for understanding health systems are highly influenced by the history of institutions in the advanced market economies.* This means their transferability is questionable. Second, *the regulation of health systems in advanced market economies has precluded the development of certain other types of organization which may be equally or more effective.* This means that low and middle-income countries may be in a better position to innovate institutionally. Third, *the regulatory arrangements in the advanced market economies strongly influence international standards and the development of health systems in other countries.* However, this does not mean that the direction of development of global health systems is already determined. The rapid growth of demand for health-related goods and services and the emergence of a variety of organizations to meet this demand have created opportunities for major changes in the organization of both national and global markets. Thus, policies and interventions over the next few years are likely to influence the path of development of these market systems for many years to come (Bloom and Standing, 2008).

Health systems in low- and middle-income countries

National health systems in developing countries reflect different historical legacies. Most countries have long-established health-related markets based on different medical knowledge systems and embedded in 'traditional' institutional arrangements. During the second half of the twentieth century, anti-colonial and/or post-revolutionary governments in much of Africa and Asia attempted to provide equitable access to 'modern' health services for all. Strategies for achieving this aim were influenced by a shared understanding of development as a state-led process for creating the building blocks of a modern economy. Many governments constructed a network of basic health facilities, trained and deployed health workers, established drug distribution systems and created vertically organized public health programmes. There was little interest in the previously established health markets, and their importance diminished in many countries.

The subsequent history of national health systems has varied greatly (Bloom and Standing, 2008). Some countries have established and sustained well-organized government health services, but health services in many others have evolved into pluralistic health systems with large informal markets. Some have experienced shocks such as war and civil disturbance, natural disasters, prolonged economic crisis and the pandemic of HIV and AIDS, which have eroded the financial basis of the public health system and led to changes in the attitudes and behaviour of government employees. Much economic activity in these countries occurs outside the organized economy. The health sector has mirrored these changes with a rapid spread of markets into services previously organized through 'traditional' relationships or by the state. Other countries, including many transition economies and other countries that are encouraging the growth of markets, have substantially altered the balance between the state and markets. Some are well on the way to becoming advanced market economies. Others have experienced substantial economic decline and resemble those described above. Still others have experienced rapid economic growth and concomitant increase in market-oriented activities in health.

Implications for markets and states

Private providers in advanced market economies operate within a highly regulated context. The situation is quite different in countries where the legal framework established to support a state-led health system remains intact and government health workers generally have contracts that imply they are in full-time employment, yet in practice they rely on market-like activities to maintain their income. Some 'public' health services could more accurately be described as publicly subsidized markets, with a number of regulatory rigidities and where the gap between formal employment contracts and long-established reality provides anomalous incentives for health workers. Informal providers, and public-sector employees who receive informal payments, may operate outside any legal framework, and there is limited capacity to enforce regulations because of a lack of resources, inadequate understanding by regulators of their role or because they have little incentive to act (Ensor and Weinzierl, 2006). Indeed, regulators may have strong incentives not to enforce regulations. There are often large discontinuities between the legal framework and the real social and economic relationships. In many cases the health system is highly segmented, with the better-off benefiting from institutions such as health insurance and a relatively effective regulatory framework, while the poor rely largely on informal markets.

The recognition that much market activity takes place outside a formal regulatory framework and that public systems are increasingly involved in formal and informal markets suggests that the clear demarcation between private and public sectors in advanced market economies does not necessarily apply elsewhere (Bloom *et al.*, 2009). The definition of the private sector by Smith *et al.* (2001) as 'those who work outside the direct control of the state' raises big questions. For example, how does one define government-owned health facilities in China, which generate a high proportion of their revenue from payments by patients? How should one regard government employees in other countries who rely on informal payments to earn a living, or work part of their day in 'private' facilities?

Categorization of organizations in terms of ownership and legal status is similarly problematic. For example, a recent report on private health systems in Africa differentiated between for-profit providers, not-for-profit organizations (including faith-based organizations) and social enterprises (International Finance Corporation, 2007). The meaning of these categories is clear in countries with highly developed regulatory frameworks that provide different patterns of incentive to each type of organization. That is not the case in many African countries, where it may be difficult to differentiate between the incentives that managers and employees of 'for-profit' and some 'not-for-profit' organizations face. Performance may differ greatly between health facilities that notionally share the same mission (Tibandebage and Mackintosh, 2005). We need to move beyond a simple public–private dichotomy to develop a more nuanced understanding of markets and the influence of the state and other agencies on their performance. As Das *et al.* (2008) note, the performance of both public and private providers of health services is strongly influenced by the incentives they face.

Analyses of 'government failure' in many low- and middle-income countries note that government employees do not behave like 'Weberian bureaucrats' who are paid a salary and provided with good career prospects in exchange for being public servants who act in the interest of the population. Performance is strongly influenced by financial incentives and political and patronage relationships. In many instances there is a fine line between market-like behaviour that has accrued a degree of legitimacy and behaviour that is socially understood to be corrupt (Lewis, 2006; Vian, 2008). For example, some informal payments may be regarded as 'fair' in a context of very low public-sector pay, while other payments may be viewed as exploitative. There is an equally difficult-to-define line between the use of regulatory powers for the public good and in the interest of specific stakeholders, including the regulators themselves. Interventions that do not take this reality into account can have unintended consequences (Pritchett and Woolcock, 2004).

The same factors that contribute to the failure of government systems also influence the performance of markets. North (1990) stresses the importance of agreed and enforced rules and associated expectations and behavioural norms in facilitating the effective performance of markets. In the absence of these institutions one finds major failures of both states and markets (Chang, 2007). Some current manifestations of these failures in the health sector are the growing problem of counterfeit drugs, inappropriate use of anti-microbial and anti-viral agents, and problems with the quality and cost of care.

Effective regulatory structures usually involve partnerships between the state and other stakeholders. For example, the drug regulatory systems of the advanced market economies were established in close consultation with the pharmaceutical industry and they reflect a balance between public and stakeholder interests (Abraham, 1995). Some argue that the balance has favoured powerful stakeholders, but most agree that some form of regulatory partnership is needed. In contrast, the governments of many low-income countries have tried to create these structures without direct involvement of industry actors. And large international companies have taken little responsibility for the use of their products in export markets. The result has often been weakly regulated health markets, both nationally and internationally. One encouraging response has been the emergence of regulatory partnerships ('co-production') between government and other actors (Joshi and Moore, 2004). Although these regulatory arrangements are subject to the influence of narrow interests, they also reflect recognition that these actors have a shared interest in the creation of a trusted and effective health system.

Markets and the health knowledge economy

A number of propositions about health systems and markets lie at the core of this book:

- The reality of healthcare systems in many developing economies is of high levels of marketization, pluralistic provision and a large gap between the goal of a functioning publicly provided and regulated health system and the messy reality that confronts both users and providers. We argue for better analytical and practical understanding of this reality. It is an argument not for privatization but for creative thinking on how to start from this reality in constructing health systems that work much better for the poor.
- Health systems are frequently highly segmented. This is no longer just a financial segmentation, in which the better-off either can afford to pay for good-quality care or are protected by privileged financing arrangements such as private insurance, leaving the poor to underfunded public health systems. Health markets increasingly dominate transactions for all socio-economic groups, as demonstrated in major changes in health-seeking behaviour. Markets themselves are segmented in complex ways that reflect their users' purchasing power (or lack of it), their cultural and social needs, understandings of health and disease, and assessments of provider reputation.

- The development of trust-based institutional arrangements that provide a reasonable guarantee of competence and effectiveness has lagged behind this growth in market-type relationships. However, the path dependency of health systems means that institutional pathways to more equitable health systems are likely to take different forms outside the Organisation for Economic Co-operation and Development (OECD) countries. These forms will reflect the different development pathways, sets of actors and existing and emerging institutional arrangements, including 'informal' ones, in a particular country.
- The form these institutional arrangements take, including the role of government, reflects a country's political economy. Moreover, a regime's legitimacy can be affected by the perceived safety, effectiveness and fairness of the health sector.
- Information asymmetry pervades health markets and is considered to be a key market failure in health. This can particularly disadvantage the poor, who lack both financial and *knowledge-based* access to competent, affordable health care. We argue that information asymmetry pervades all knowledge-based market transactions, not only those concerned with health. There is thus much to be learned from different market sectors on other kinds of approaches to reducing information asymmetries in ways that benefit the poor.
- Recent developments in information and communications technology and the development of very large organizations that function as knowledge inter-mediaries are creating major new opportunities for structuring access to expert knowledge and influencing the behaviour of providers and users of health-related goods and services.

Understanding market systems

This subsection builds on these core propositions to examine in more detail how health-related markets operate. Their role is to make widely available the benefits of expert medical knowledge, in terms of advice and treatment and embodied in goods such as pharmaceuticals. It is important to clarify that this analysis does not equate a market with the delivery of a (commercial) service but refers to the whole set of supporting functions and rules enacted by different sets of players ('public' and 'private') at different stages of the delivery, hence the use of the term 'market system'. Along with financing mechanisms to provide equitable access, efficient operation of these markets depends on the provision of effective ways to address information asymmetry. This involves setting and enforcement of rules and provision of accurate and timely information. Health systems tend to have complex arrangements for achieving these functions. How they operate in a specific social context is key to understanding how performance incentives and disincentives will play out.

A recent body of work focuses on how markets in countries with less developed formal institutions can be made to work better for poor people (DFID and SDC, 2008; Elliot *et al.*, 2008). It emphasizes the crucial role that markets play in mediating relationships between providers and users of goods and services, and

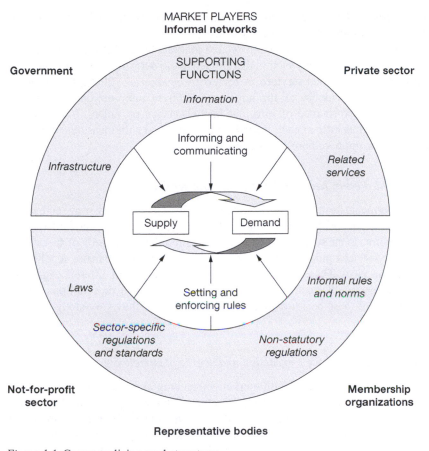

MARKET PLAYERS
Informal networks

Government

SUPPORTING
FUNCTIONS

Private sector

Information

Infrastructure

Informing and
communicating

*Related
services*

Supply | Demand

Laws

Setting and
enforcing rules

*Informal rules
and norms*

*Sector-specific
regulations
and standards*

*Non-statutory
regulations*

**Not-for-profit
sector**

**Membership
organizations**

Representative bodies

Figure 1.1 Conceptualizing market systems.

Source: Adapted from Elliot *et al.* (2008: figure 3).

argues that it is important to understand them as complex *systems* which can perform well or badly.

Figure 1.1 illustrates the multiple and interrelated institutions that influence market function. At the centre are the exchanges between providers and consumers of the relevant goods and services. These exchanges are governed by the interplay of formal and informal rules, whose establishment and enforcement involve actors who in turn are influenced by a variety of factors. Supporting functions provide an environment within which the performance of market players may be enhanced or constrained. This environment also includes multiple actors and organizations, legal regulations, and the norms and values of suppliers and users of goods and services. Given these interactions between the different elements of a market system, Elliot *et al.* (2008) argue that interventions that focus too narrowly on specific aspects, for example strengthening the management of a given organization or changing particular macroeconomic policies, are likely to fail. Reforms need to bridge the micro, meso and macro levels in building institutions that contribute to improved market performance.

Recent efforts to influence health-related markets have illustrated the need to take into account the many factors that influence the performance of providers of health-related goods and services. A review by Shah *et al.* (2010), for example, summarizes the evidence on the impact of different interventions intended to improve the performance of informal health service providers. It found that training alone has little impact; it needs to be combined with measures to provide incentives for improved prescribing practices.

Types of markets in health-related goods and services

Markets permeate health systems in complex ways. 'Upstream', they are embedded in research and development of drugs and vaccines, for example; they interface at different points in the supply chain, for instance through the provision of specialized knowledge services and innovation. 'Downstream', they are also major suppliers of goods and services. These may be simple or complex, and with different degrees of connectedness to other markets. There are no simple sets of prescriptions for the organization of these health-related market systems and they vary along multiple dimensions.

Different types of service transaction and degree of complexity

It is misleading to discuss health markets in general, as if the provision of all of them will require a single type of organization (Chakraborty and Harding, 2002; Leonard, 2000; Van Damme *et al.*, 2008). The treatment of a minor ailment, for example, may simply involve the provision of access to good-quality drugs and widely available knowledge, and may be best left to competitive markets. The management of a chronic, progressive disease requires quite high levels of trust in the advice of service providers and a willingness to make changes to lifestyle or comply with drug treatments. Major surgical treatment requires high levels of trust and expertise, and a well-organized hospital. The consequences of a failure to ensure safety and effectiveness range from mild to severe. The institutional arrangements to encourage good performance will not be the same for different types of service. The studies in this volume focus on relatively basic services used by the poor, including outpatient treatment of malaria in Nigeria and diabetes in Cambodia, sexual and reproductive health services in Bangladesh, and basic outpatient services in Bangladesh and China.

Segmented health systems

The analysis of health market systems in countries with major structural inequalities needs to take into account how different subsystems affect different social groups, including the poor. Some interventions may target the immediate needs of the poor and others may aim at a longer-term impact as knowledge of them grows, costs fall and the delivery of services spreads to poor localities. Other interventions may be too expensive for the poor and their overall impact may be to reinforce the segmentation of health-related markets, with a deleterious impact on the poor. For example, a decision to restrict all eye surgery to hospital-based specialist surgeons would deny most poor people access to low-cost cataract operations. The same applies to many regulations that reserve the provision of services to highly qualified professionals and effectively leave the providers of services to the poor unregulated and outside the law.

Ownership, mission and accountability of different market players

The categorization of market players in terms of their ownership, assumed mission and accountability requirements may not be clear-cut in countries without developed market-related institutions. There may be blurred boundaries between public and private health service providers and between 'for profit' and 'not-for-profit' organizations. There is little systematic information on the pattern of incentives that managers and employees of different types of organization face or their likely response to alternative organizational arrangements. Similarly, while there are likely to be formal accountability arrangements, it is often informal ones that determine incentives and outcomes. For instance, there may be tacit arrangements over which informal payments can be demanded and who shares in them.

Interconnected markets

The provision of medical services involves a series of interconnected markets for different goods and services. Where the patterns of incentives in one market are not aligned with the interests of the poor, other markets will be affected. Making health markets work better for the poor will often entail the need to address a problem in an interconnected or secondary market. For example, Chapter 4 (by Rahman and Agarwal) in this volume describes how the informal drug sellers in Bangladesh are strongly influenced by the large numbers of representatives of drug wholesalers, who have strong incentives to sell expensive products.

Local, national and international market systems

It is difficult to put a boundary around a market system. Some markets are mostly influenced by local, largely informal, institutional arrangements. For many others there is an interaction between local, national and international organizations and institutions. It is important to understand the links between national and global value chains (Gereffi *et al.*, 2005; Smith, 2004; Woodward, 2005). For example, the organization of the global pharmaceutical sector strongly influences the performance of local markets through arrangements to regulate quality, protect intellectual property and promote the use of new products. International service delivery organizations, including large NGOs, play an important and growing role in many countries, as do large consultancy firms and donor agencies that finance health services. The rapid emergence of branded private hospital chains as a source of high-quality medical care and of medical tourism is another example of the interaction between national and transnational markets (Chee, 2008). Global value chains in the health sector are changing rapidly, and measures to improve the performance of local markets will increasingly entail attention to supranational supply chains as they alter the patterns of incentives in local health markets.

What do institutional arrangements in health market systems do?

One way to understand the role of institutional arrangements in health and other sectors is as a means to foster 'social contracts' between actors (Bloom *et al.*, 2008). These contracts embody the expectations necessary for the establishment and maintenance of trust-based relationships and they reflect broader understandings in a given society of expected social reciprocity. In relation to health care, they enable people to purchase drugs without worrying about their safety and efficacy, and to consult possessors of medical knowledge with confidence in their expertise and ethics. They also make possible the establishment of insurance schemes to which people contribute money in the expectation that they will have support should they fall ill in the future.

These relationships also reflect and, to some extent, reinforce relationships of power. For example, in many countries the organized medical profession strongly opposes measures to improve the performance of non-professional providers mostly used by the poor (Dussault, 2008). Large pharmaceutical companies often oppose measures that threaten their markets. Markets are frequently segmented, with actors that serve different social groups following different rules and behavioural norms. Institutional arrangements are always negotiated in relation to these realities. Strategies to alter the performance of market systems must be based on an assessment of the political and social context and identification of significant power relationships between actors (Bloom, 2001).

In most countries the performance of health-related markets has broader social and political consequences, consequences that mandate institutional actions. The legitimacy of a regime is linked, to some extent, to its ability to protect the population against major health-related challenges. Scandals about counterfeit drugs, contaminated blood, inadequate responses to disease outbreaks and the impoverishment of households due to high healthcare costs can have a big political impact. Their effect will grow as countries become increasingly integrated into the global economy and local scandals influence the reputation of companies seeking global markets in pharmaceuticals or health-related services.

Institutional arrangements perform a range of functions in health systems, including reducing information asymmetries. Their overarching function is *the creation of conditions for trust in the competence and ethics of providers*. Trust is essential to the effective performance of health systems (Gilson, 2003). Users also need to feel confident that money they contribute in taxes or contributions to insurance schemes will entitle them to receive care when they need it, sometimes years later. In the absence of such confidence, users may have to invest a great deal of effort to find a competent provider or forgo the potential benefits of health-care technologies. The other side of the social contract between providers and users of health-related goods and services is the reputation of providers. Providers need to believe that they will benefit from a reputation for skill and ethical behaviour in terms of income, future career prospects, social status and influence.

Institutional arrangements are a critical factor in *building the legitimacy of health system governance and change*. The sustainability of institutional arrangements and the expectation of compliance with rules depend on the degree to which they are perceived to be legitimate. This goes beyond the reputation of a specific facility or organization. It is related to the degree to which the rules are perceived by the population more generally to address major problems, take into account the needs of different social groups and command widespread consent. One major challenge is the balance between the interests of specific stakeholders and an agreed public interest. In some contexts it may only be possible to build a consensus around a very small core of particularly important regulatory issues.

Creating institutional arrangements for more orderly health-related markets

Service providers have evolved several strategies for building a reputation for expertise and ethical behaviour (Montagu, 2002; Mills *et al.*, 2002; Prata *et al.*, 2005). People are often willing to pay a premium to service providers that have a good reputation. These strategies largely evolved in sectors such as financial services, restaurants and hotels, but they are being adopted in the health sector. Formal approaches include:

- The development of services through large, well-known organizations, such as NGOs, hospital chains and retail pharmacy chains, which have an incentive to protect their reputation through internal management systems.
- The establishment of franchises, in which franchisees agree to adhere to certain standards in order to trade with a particular brand name.
- The accreditation or licensing of a facility or provider by an independent agency. This may be a national accreditation body, a professional licensing agency, a trade association or one of a variety of other types of trusted national or local organizations.

A growing number of initiatives around the world have applied different elements of these approaches to health-related goods and services. Chapter 9 in this volume (by Champion *et al.*) reviews the available evidence on the impact of these approaches on the provision of health services. Informal mechanisms for building trust and reputation, based on local networks, are as important as, or more important than, these other approaches in many contexts. Cross and MacGregor (2010) summarize the contributions of anthropological studies to an understanding of the institutional context within which informal providers are embedded. The chapters in this volume by Oladepo and Lucas, and Iqbal *et al.* (Chapters 7 and 3) show how a combination of linking to local accountability structures and involving associations of informal providers themselves can begin to provide a mechanism through which providers of services can build a reputation for good practice.

The flow of knowledge and information is vitally important to the performance of health-related markets. Both providers and users, including many of the poor, increasingly live in a world where multiple sources of information are available. The chapter by Lucas (Chapter 10) discusses the opportunities and challenges associated with the rapid development of ICTs. This proliferation of sources of expert knowledge has created a new need for trusted knowledge brokers and new initiatives to fill this growing gap. A number of initiatives disseminate information on performance through citizens' report cards, publication of achievement of performance targets and establishment of citizen complaint lines. Consumer associations play an increasingly important role in some countries (Peters and Muraleedharan, 2008).

The lack of a strong regulatory state at different levels has created a vacuum into which other actors are stepping to provide some kind of market order. This often involves a partnership with the national or local state to co-produce regulation (Joshi and Moore, 2004; Peters and Muraleedharan, 2008). These partnerships may involve private companies, business associations, professions and community or citizen groups. These raise important questions about how 'public interest' is constructed out of this complexity of interests and which sets of actors dominate in this process. One of the big unanswered questions about the development of health market systems is *what are the relative roles that local, national and global reputations and actors will play?* This will depend on the balance of local, national and global interests involved and the degree to which governments and international bodies can implement effective regulatory arrangements that go beyond the level of the local.

Understanding and theorizing from local realities

The remainder of the book combines case studies in several countries and desk-based reviews of evidence. Chapter 2 (by Kanjilal and Mazumdar) presents an overview of the changing relationships between the state and markets in India's health sector and highlights the many new challenges that policy-makers face. The chapters by Iqbal *et al.* (Chapter 3), Rahman and Agarwal (Chapter 4) and Bloom *et al.* (Chapter 5) present locality-specific case studies of the operation of the markets for general outpatient services in Bangladesh and China. The next three chapters present case studies of markets for specific health-related services: Standing *et al.* focus on sexual and reproductive health services in Bangladesh, Oladepo and Lucas on malaria treatment in Nigeria and Van Pelt *et al.* on the treatment of diabetes in Cambodia. These six chapters illustrate the important influence of context on the structure of health market systems and the different approaches being taken to improve their performance. The next two chapters review evidence on different aspects of health markets. Champion *et al.* in Chapter 9 summarize the evidence on the impact of alternative strategies for improving the performance of health markets, and Lucas in Chapter 10 presents evidence on the different ways that ICTs are changing health systems. Bishai and Champion in Chapter 11 present a theoretical approach for analysing the opportunities and challenges associated with adapting franchising models for improving the performance of health services providers. The final chapter presents an overview of broad ways forward and the implications for future research.

References

Abraham, J. (1995) 'Partial progress? The development of American and British drug regulation', in *Science, Politics and the Pharmaceutical Industry: Controversy and Drug Bias in Drug Regulation*, UCL Press, London

Altenstetter, C. and Busse, R. (2005) 'Health care reform in Germany: patchwork change within established governance structures', *Journal of Health Politics, Policy and Law*, 30 (1–2): 121–142

Bennett, S., McPake, B. and Mills, A. (1997) *Private Health Providers in Developing Countries*, Zed Press, London

Bloom, G. (2001) 'Equity in health in unequal societies: meeting health needs in contexts of social change', *Health Policy*, 57 (3): 205–224

Bloom, G. and Standing, H. (2001) 'Pluralism and marketisation in the health sector: meeting health needs in contexts of social change in low and middle income countries', IDS Working Paper no. 136, IDS, Brighton

Bloom, G. and Standing, H. (2008) 'Future health systems: why future? Why now?', *Social Science and Medicine*, 66 (10): 2067–2075

Bloom, G., Standing, H. and Lloyd, R. (2008) 'Markets, information asymmetry and health care: towards new social contracts', *Social Science and Medicine*, 66 (10): 2076–2087

Bloom, G., Champion, C., Lucas, H., Peters, D. and Standing, H. (2009) 'Making health markets work better for poor people: improving provider performance', Future Health Systems Working Paper no. 6. Online, available at: www.futurehealthsystems.org/storage/publications/working-papers/wp6.pdf

Chakraborty, S. and Harding, A. (2002) 'Conducting a private health sector assessment', in A. Harding and A. Preker (eds) *Private Participation in Health Services Handbook*, World Bank, Washington, DC

Chang, H. J. (2007) 'Understanding the relationship between institutions and economic development: some key theoretical issues', in H. J. Chang (ed.) *Institutional Change and Economic Development*, Anthem Press, London

Chee, H. L. (2008) 'Ownership, control and contention: challenges for the future of healthcare in Malaysia', *Social Science and Medicine*, 66 (10): 2145–2156

Cross, J. and MacGregor, H. (2010) 'Knowledge, legitimacy and economic practice in informal markets for medicine: a critical review of research', *Social Science and Medicine*, 71: 1593–1600

Das, J., Hammer, J. and Leonard, K. (2008) 'The quality of medical advice in low-income countries', *Journal of Economic Perspectives*, 22 (2): 93–114

David, P. A. (1985) 'Clio and the economics of QWERTY', *American Economic Review*, 75 (2): 332–337

DFID and SDC (2008) *A Synthesis of the Making Markets Work for the Poor (M4P) Approach*, Department for International Development, London; Swiss Agency for Development and Cooperation, Berne

Dussault, G. (2008) 'The health professions and the performance of health systems in low income countries: support or obstacle', *Social Science and Medicine*, 66 (10): 2088–2095

Elliot, D., Gibson, A. and Hitchins, R. (2008) 'Making markets work for the poor: rationale and practice', *Enterprise Development and Microfinance*, 19 (2): 101–119

Ensor, T. and Weinzierl, S. (2006) *A Review of Regulation in the Health Sector in Low and Middle Income Countries: Signposts to More Effective States*, Institute of Development Studies, Brighton

Gereffi, G. (1994) 'The organization of buyer-driven global commodity chains: how U.S. retailers shape overseas production networks', in G. Gereffi and M. Korzeniewicz (eds) *Commodity Chains and Global Capitalism*, Praeger, London

Gereffi, G., Humphrey, J. and Sturgeon, T. (2005) 'The governance of global value chains', *Review of International Political Economy*, 12 (1): 78–104

Gilson, L. (2003) 'Trust and the development of health care as a social institution', *Social Science and Medicine*, 56 (7): 1453–1468

Gordon, C. (2005) *Dead on Arrival: The Politics of Health Care in Twentieth-Century America*, Princeton University Press, Princeton, NJ

International Finance Corporation (2007) *The Business of Health in Africa*, World Bank Group, IFC Health and Education Department, Washington, DC. Online, available at: www.ifc.org/ifcext/healthinafrica.nsf/Content/FullReport

Joshi, A. and Moore, M. (2004) 'Institutionalised co-production: unorthodox public service delivery in challenging environments', *Journal of Development Studies*, 40 (4): 31–49

Leonard, D. (2000) 'Lessons from the new institutional economics for the structural reform of human health services in Africa', in D. Leonard (ed.) *Africa's Changing Markets for Health and Veterinary Services*, Macmillan, Basingstoke, UK

Lewis, N. (2006) 'Governance and corruption in public health care systems', Center for Global Development Working Paper 76, Center for Global Development, Washington, DC

Mackintosh, M. and Koivusalo, M. (2005) 'Health systems and commercialization: in search of good sense', in M. Mackintosh and M. Koivusalo (eds) *Commercialization of Health Care: Global and Local Dynamics and Policy Responses*, Palgrave Macmillan, Basingstoke, UK

Mills, A., Brugha, R., Hanson, K. and McPake, B. (2002) 'What can be done about the private health sector in low-income countries?', *Bulletin of the World Health Organization*, 80 (4): 325–330

Montagu, D. (2002) 'Franchising of health services in developing countries', *Health Policy and Planning*, 17 (2): 121–130

National Health Accounts (2007) Summaries of country data. Online, available from: www.who.int/nha/country/en

North, D. C. (1990) *Institutions, Institutional Change and Economic Performance*, Cambridge University Press, New York

Peters, D. H. and Muraleedharan, V. (2008) 'Regulating India's health services: to what end? What future?', *Social Science and Medicine*, 66 (10): 2133–2144

Piersen, P. and Skocpol, T. (2002) 'Historical institutionalism in contemporary political science', in I. Katznelson and H. V. Milner (eds) *Political Science: The State of the Discipline*, W. W. Norton, New York

Prata, N., Montagu, D. and Jefferys, E. (2005) 'Private sector, human resources and health franchising in Africa', *Bulletin of the World Health Organization*, 83: 274–279

Pritchett, L. and Woolcock, M. (2004) 'Solutions when the solution is the problem: arraying the disarray in development', *World Development*, 32 (2): 191–212

Rochaix, L. and Wilsford, D. (2005) 'State autonomy, policy paralysis: paradoxes of institutions and culture in the French health care system', *Journal of Health Politics Policy and Law*, 30 (1–2): 97–120

Shah, N. M., Brieger, W. R. and Peters, D. H. (2010) 'Can interventions improve health services from private providers in low and middle-income countries? A comprehensive review of the literature', *Health Policy and Planning*. doi:10.1093/heapol/czq074

Smith, E., Brugha, R. and Zwi, A. (2001) *Working with Private Sector Providers for Better Health Care*, Options Consultancy, London

Smith, R. D. (2004) 'Foreign direct investment and trade in health services: a review of the literature', *Social Science and Medicine*, 59: 2313–2323

Thelen, K. (2003) 'How institutions evolve: insights from comparative historical analysis', in J. Mahoney and D. Rueschemeyer (eds) *Comparative Historical Analysis in the Social Sciences*, Cambridge University Press, Cambridge

Tibandebage, P. and Mackintosh, M. (2005) 'The market shaping of charges, trust and abuse: health care transactions in Tanzania', *Social Science and Medicine*, 61: 1385–1396

Van Damme, W., Kober, K. and Kegels, G. (2008) 'Scaling-up antiretroviral treatment in Southern African countries with human resource shortage: how will health systems adapt?', *Social Science and Medicine*, 66 (10): 2108–2122

Vian, T. (2008) 'Review of corruption in the health sector: theory, methods and interventions', *Health Policy and Planning*, 23: 83–94

Woodward, D. (2005) 'The GATS and trade in health services: implications for health care in developing countries', *Review of International Political Economy*, 12 (3): 511–534

2 Transition in the Indian healthcare market

Barun Kanjilal and Sumit Mazumdar

Background

The Indian healthcare market has been passing through an unprecedented transitional phase in recent years, bringing forth new questions for health and public policy. The transition is integrated with the fast-track economic growth that was triggered in the early 1990s, and took a sharp upward turn under the wrap of a macroeconomic structural adjustment programme and associated neo-liberal policies. The reform process was targeted to unshackle the economy from commands, controls and restrictions on private investment and to correct for internal and external macroeconomic disequilibria, which led to a severe crisis in public finance and international trade at the beginning of the 1990s. In other words, the main goals were to allow market forces to stabilize the economy, spur economic growth and integrate the local economy to the global marketplace.

As expected, the Indian health sector responded to the economic reforms with several visible signs that were manifested in two distinct ways. First, there were attempts to reposition the government's role in the health sector in the new paradigm of liberalized growth. Government spending on health as a percentage of GDP declined through the 1990s (Peters *et al.*, 2002), and a few states initiated a cautious process of health-sector reform, with support by the World Bank and other development agencies. In addition, user fees were introduced in the health sector in many states (Qadeer, 2000; Purohit, 2001). The second process, running in parallel and inspired primarily by general economic reforms, manifested itself in automatic market responses such as increased flow of private investments to the health sector. This process set off a rapid proliferation of the private sector, leading to a rapidly expanding healthcare sector growing at a compound annual turnover rate of 16 per cent during the 1990s, coupled with an equally impressive growth in employment (PricewaterhouseCoopers, 2007).

Historically, public health interventions in India until the 1990s were guided by a vision of a vertically integrated and publicly provided universal healthcare system (Peters *et al.*, 2002). Consequently, a vast network of primary, secondary and tertiary health facilities were rolled out across the country during the period. A number of vertical programmes to control vector-borne and infectious diseases and to promote universal immunization were introduced. However, the vision gradually turned into mere rhetoric or a 'utopian appeal' since the country's public investment in the health system had been too small (less than 1 per cent of GDP) to translate the vision into a reality (Peters *et al.*, 2002). Even the available funds failed to promise much, owing to typical inefficiencies in financing, provision, organization and regulation by the public sector.

Against this dismal backdrop, the new economic regime pushed neo-liberal policies leading to rapid proliferation of the private sector in the Indian health market. As a result, modern clinical procedures and new medical technologies and drugs have become available, leading to a huge expansion of consumer choice. With market forces sweeping across, economics rather than ideology guides the changing structure, pattern and complexities of the healthcare market. From the demand side, an expanding middle class with more disposable income to purchase healthcare fuels the process.

The glowing face of reform, however, is counterbalanced by a set of unintended adverse consequences. Increasing commodification of health care is an unavoidable result of the marketization process, which has serious equity implications, especially in a country like India which has a highly heterogeneous consumer base and unequal ability to pay (Wilson, 2010). Recent Indian evidence shows that transition to a marketized system of health care, without adequate social protection and appropriate regulatory arrangements, underpins a significant risk of producing distorted markets and a new set of vulnerabilities, inequalities and health-related poverty (Garg and Karan, 2005; Berman *et al.*, 2010).

The complex linkages and structural features that characterize the contemporary transition in the Indian healthcare market make it imperative to delineate the underlying processes and expected fallout of such phenomena. The broad questions to address for decoding the complexities are:

- Transition in the structure and spread of the market – how, to what extent and why has the market changed during economic reforms?
- Linkages, responses and impact – how are the market players affected and how did they respond to these changes? What are the welfare consequences from the social perspective?
- Institutional arrangements – how and to what extent have the institutional arrangements changed to influence and regulate the marketization process?

This chapter examines the pathways of transition in the Indian healthcare market by addressing the above three issues in the context of three key output components (or sub-markets) of curative health care. The markets for: (1) inpatient care; (2) outpatient care; and (3) pharmaceutical products and services. It is important to break down the analysis of the market as a whole since the marketization process, as explained later, has quite diverse impacts on various sub-markets. The rationale behind the selection of these three markets is that these three components comprehensively reflect the maximum effects of the marketization process in the Indian health sector because of their direct links with the consumers. The major issues we raise and answer include the changing comparative roles of private providers in healthcare services, emergence of new market linkages (e.g. pharmaceuticals and medical technologies) and the consequent aspects of regulation and welfare of the market transitions in terms of rising costs to the consumers. We draw extensively on extant literature, industry reports and market analyses, available national health survey data, and the research evidence from Future Health Systems (FHS) – a research programme consortium of global institutions from several countries, including India.

Inpatient care: corporatization of health care

Transition in structure and spread

Empirical evidence strongly suggests a consistently rising market share of private providers during the past two decades in the Indian inpatient care market. Data from national healthcare surveys carried out by the National Sample Survey Organisation (NSSO) during the period 1986–2004,[1] which can be roughly classified as pre-reform, early-reform and late-reform years (with respect to the initiation of structural adjustment processes in 1991), reveal that for curative care requiring hospitalization, the share of private hospitals – in terms of percentage of hospitalized cases – increased from 40 per cent in 1986 to about 62 per cent in 2004 for urban users, and to 58 per cent for rural users (Figure 2.1). Only in a very few of the major states (West Bengal, Orissa, Rajasthan and Madhya Pradesh) was reliance on public hospitals found to be proportionately higher. By contrast, in most of the economically developed states (e.g. Gujarat, Maharashtra, Punjab and Karnataka) only about a quarter of all hospitalized cases were registered in public hospitals.

The gradual and steady ascension of the private sector to the dominant position in the inpatient care market is also confirmed by supply-side evidence. For

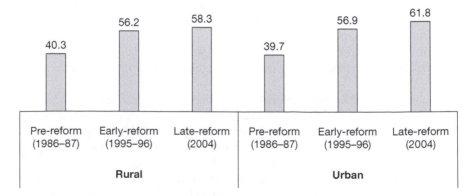

Figure 2.1 Utilization of private health facilities for hospitalized ailments: India, 1986–2004.

Source: NSSO (forty-second, fifty-second and sixtieth round).

example, the share of the private sector in the total number of beds in the country has gradually increased from 41 per cent in 1983 to an estimated 78 per cent in 2009 (Bhandari and Gupta, 2010). However, most of these beds belong to small-scale private hospitals (those with 5–30 beds) owned and run by a single proprietorship or partnership (Muraleedharan and Nandraj, 2003).

Parallel to the consolidation of a predominant position of the private sector in an increasingly commercialized inpatient care market, a number of other developments have been taking place during the past few years. These include a vibrant growth in tertiary and super-speciality care that has brought in corporate houses, venture capital and a spate of mergers and acquisitions leading to a 'corporatization' of the market. Accounting for about 10 per cent of the private hospitals, corporate hospitals (owned and managed by corporate listed companies and distinct from proprietorship or partnership enterprises), which include reputable concerns such as Apollo Hospitals, Fortis, Max, Escorts, Wockhardt, Reliance, Aditya Birla Group, etc., have entered the market during the past decade and have since been engaged in ambitious expansion plans (IBEF, 2010). After consolidating their bases in highly urbanized metro cities and introducing the concept of 'brand equity', the corporate players have targeted the non-metro and smaller cities, demonstrating the rule of vertical integration of service delivery and inducing tough competition with local non-corporate service providers. Their expansion is often facilitated and subsidized by favourable public policies such as tax exemption and subsidy of land prices, and the limited regulatory barriers to entry in the market.

Emerging healthcare segments like diagnostic chains, medical device manufacturers as well as hospital chains are increasingly attracting investments from a variety of venture capitalists, with private equity funding predicted to rise from US$14.8 billion in 2006–2007 to US$33.6 billion in 2012 (IBEF, 2009). Attracted by a gradual relaxation of foreign investment norms and several inducements being on offer, foreign direct investment (FDI) in the healthcare sector has also been on the rise. During the period 2000–2009, an amount of US$1,707.52 million was pumped into the drugs and pharmaceutical sector, and an additional US$786.14 million into hospitals and diagnostic centres, together accounting for 2.2 per cent of the net FDI inflows in the country (DIPP, 2010). The market for medical diagnostics and technologies appears to be the hotspot for both domestic and foreign investments and is projected to contribute US$2.5 billion to the healthcare industry by 2012. The market has also witnessed strong interest among the key corporate players for upcoming health Special Economic Zones (SEZs) and 'Health Cities', with current pipeline projects for the latter reaching a committed investment of about US$ 20 billion (IBEF, 2009). A related ancillary sector of medical tourism is seen as having high growth potential, partly because of the increased costs of treatments in developed countries and growing adherence to global accreditation norms by corporate hospitals in the country. Medical tourism is expected to generate revenue of US$2.4 billion by 2012, growing at a compound annual growth rate (CAGR) of over 27 per cent during the period 2009–2012. The number of medical tourists is anticipated to grow at a CAGR of over 19 per cent in the forecast period to reach 1.1 million by 2012 (IBEF, 2010).

Linkages, responses and impacts

The shake-up in the private hospital market has had some significant knock-on effects on several related stakeholders in the inpatient care market. For example, 'quality of care', often perceived as the core strength of private hospitals, has become a buzzword even among the public providers, for whom quality was hardly on their agenda in the past. Many states are introducing quality accreditation standards for all government hospitals, although the results are yet to be visible in terms of improvement in patient outcomes or impact on the population. The drive towards better quality standards in government hospitals reflects a forced orientation of the public sector to respond to market demand for better quality.

Apart from quality, the government's response has been reflected in three areas: (1) creating an enabling environment for the entry and growth of private investment in the hospital sector, (2) building partnerships with for-profit private players in providing hospital services through various public–private partnership (PPP) models, and (3) participating in the market as an active player to generate additional resources for government hospitals. The initiative for enabling this environment resulted in a series of input subsidies (such as allotment of land for hospitals at concessional prices and subsidy for investment in medical equipment) and fiscal incentives (e.g. exemption from local levies and sales taxes for investment in medical equipment) (Purohit, 2001). The PPP models, adopted by several states, allowed conditional entry of private investors in the provision of non-clinical services (such as cleaning and waste management) and supporting services (such as diagnostic services) in government hospitals. The third area, generation of internal resources, primarily included introducing user fees at secondary- and tertiary-level government hospitals.

The responses of the public sector indicate an inclination to engage in the marketization process; however, they fail to reflect a clear strategy on how to internalize the public sector's redefined role within the boundary of traditional principles of a welfare state and a set of ambitious public health goals set by the National Health Policy.[2] Without such a strategy, the responses from the policymakers at the state level look weak, inadequate and often directionless. For example, the input and fiscal incentives have helped the private hospitals congregate only in urban areas, where patients can pay, at the expense of rural areas, where they cannot. Similarly, the unchanged incentive structure for the human resources in government hospitals coupled with a fast-growing private sector helps distort the market linkages where the government doctors are often found to act as agents of private hospitals.

The implication for users, however, is more significant. Because of the weak presence of any social protection or risk-pooling mechanisms, almost all of the private cost of treatment is shifted to the users, pushing India into the highest-ranked category in terms of the share of out-of-pocket health spending (OOPS) in total health expenditure (about 76 per cent). The burden of OOPS is disproportionately higher in private hospitals compared to their government counterparts. For example, in 2004, hospitalization would have required a rural user of a private hospital to spend Rs 7,408 on average, which is more than double the amount a user of a public hospital would have had to spend (Rs 3,238) (NSSO, 2004). The drift is much more prominent in urban areas, where a private client would have spent about three times as much as a public client (Rs 11,533 and Rs 3,877 respectively). Given that the share of private hospitals has further increased and the cost of treatment has multiplied since 2004, the market has a significant, and sometimes catastrophic, impact on the economy of a large number of Indian households. The numbers of households falling below the poverty line (BPL) as a result of inpatient care, as found in a recent paper (Berman *et al.*, 2010), is astoundingly high (2.46 million, or 1.3 per cent of households), implying that at least one household in a hundred is silently marching towards poverty every year as a result of inpatient care. Most of these households are expected to be users of private hospitals since, as a recent study shows, about 48 per cent of private users incurred catastrophically high OOPS, compared to only 15 per cent of public users (Future Health Systems, 2010).

The disproportionately high cost of inpatient care in private hospitals may be attributed to two major causes. First is the information asymmetry and absence of an effective regulatory mechanism. Control by the private hospitals of prices as well as of utilization remains conspicuously strong. Second, increasing corporatization and the consequent 'branding' initiatives have unleashed competition among hospitals to buy the latest capital-intensive technology and build more hospitable infrastructures – a process that is called a 'medical arms race' by some health policy analysts. These investments do not always justify their benefits, but they push the price up at a galloping rate. Not only have the rising costs aggravated the impoverishing impacts of private inpatient care, but also they have raised the barrier for many people, who remain untreated because private costs are prohibitive and public care is unavailable.

The entry of private insurers and their managing agents, third-party administrators (TPAs), in the Indian insurance market in the early part of the millennium – another offshoot of economic reforms – has added new dimensions to the complexities of the market. The private insurance market is unfolding along traditional paths, keeping insurers (and TPAs), hospitals and insured patients at arm's length from each other and, hence, building a relationship based on mistrust and tension. Owing to the lack of standards and regulations in India governing hospitals, nursing homes and other healthcare providers, the quality and cost of health care vary substantially across India and among service providers. While TPAs attempt to prescribe uniform fees and standards of service to avoid costly duplication in diagnostic and other customer care aspects, the service providers are resisting such moves and tend to form cartels. They have also begun to adopt dual fee schedules: a higher rate for customers preferring to get treatment under 'cashless' schemes administered through the TPAs, and a lower one for direct settlement. There are also suggestions of significant delays in settlement of bills by TPAs to healthcare providers.

Institutional arrangements

Despite rapid corporatization, the private inpatient care market remains a highly complex, heterogeneous entity, with wide variations in provider quality – technical and interpersonal, and in competence and treatment efficacy. At the macro level there are concerns regarding inequitable distribution of private hospitals and distortions in public–private relations which, as we argued earlier, remain largely unaddressed owing to failure of the public policy-makers to internalize the growth of the private sector. At the micro level, some of the main causes of concern include the potential for unnecessary services, high prices or skimping on quality (Peters and Muraleedharan, 2008).

Transition to a market economy requires appropriate institutional arrangements that would stimulate growth and regulate the market towards national health goals. The Indian story is quite blurry on this front, although there are several institutions that, taken together, could play useful roles (Bloom *et al.*, 2008).[3] However, except for judiciary and consumer courts, which have played a limited role in regulating hospital malpractices, none of the institutional players could act effectively to reduce the risks of marketization. Clearly, the spread of markets has been much faster than the capacity of the state and other key actors to establish regulatory arrangements to influence their performance, a state of affairs found in many other developing countries (Bloom *et al.*, 2011). The political response to rising hospital costs, for example, is limited to launching state-funded voluntary health insurance schemes for the poor, such as Rashtriya Swasthya Bima Yojana (RSBY), piggybacking on public and private insurance companies. The full potential of this scheme is yet to be assessed; however, recent evidence does not show any sign of its reaching all the poor in the near future (Narayana, 2010). Also, recent findings suggest that insurance schemes that cover only inpatient expenses, like RSBY, will fail to protect the poor adequately against impoverishment due to spending on health (Shahrawat and Rao, 2011).

Outpatient care: rapid spread of the underground market

Transition in structure and spread

Historically, the Indian outpatient care market has always been dominated by the private sector. The scenario did not change much in the reform period. NSSO data show that about 80 per cent of (non-hospitalized) ailing persons were treated by the private providers in 1985–1986, a proportion that remained almost as high (77 per cent) in 2004. Although the national surveys (those by the National Sample Survey Organisation, NSSO, and the National Family Health Survey, NFHS) do not classify 'private doctors' according to their qualification status, researchers and policy-makers alike concur that a large section of them belong to a category of village doctors who practise modern (i.e. allopathic) medicine without any recognized formal training or licence (Kumar *et al.*, 2007; Kanjilal *et al.*, 2008). Those belonging to this group of medical practitioners are often identified as rural medical practitioners (RMPs), or 'informal', 'unqualified', 'less than fully quali-fied' (LTFQ) providers, or simply 'quacks'. The strong presence of these providers is quite consistent with similar scenarios in developing countries, since in low-income countries one of the most striking aspects of healthcare commercializa-tion is the informalization of primary care through the creation, expansion or reinforcement of private small-scale, largely unregulated, primary provision (Mackintosh, 2003).

Future Health Systems (FHS), a research programme implemented in India during the period 2006–2010, carried out intensive research on the RMPs in the state of West Bengal and found that they had been able to establish a pivotal and ever-growing operational structure in the rural areas in the post-reform period (Kanjilal *et al.*, 2008, 2010). The structure has no legal standing, hence it may be called a 'parallel' or 'underground' market. The informality in the parallel market has its roots in the background characteristics of the providers (RMPs) and their treatment behaviour. Some of the key characteristics, as analysed by the FHS study in West Bengal, are as follows:

- About three-quarters of all RMPs did not have a college degree, and the great majority (86 per cent) had taken it up as a full-time profession. The impli-cation is that practising allopathic medicine offers a 'no-holds-barred' earning opportunity to the rural unemployed.
- Two-thirds of RMPs had past experience of working with some qualified private practitioners. This experience had helped them 'learn' the treatment path and medicines for common diseases and develop some basic skills (such as carrying out injections, checking blood pressure and even reading X-ray plates).
- Almost all of them (90 per cent) were available on call even at midnight, even though they also had been operating clinics on a normal routine.
- About 80 per cent of RMPs provided drugs with their treatments. Half of them procured these drugs from local pharmacies (the rest from wholesalers and medical representatives). Most of the RMPs (85 per cent) would sell drugs on credit or at subsidized prices if the client did not have enough cash at the point of service delivery.

What is behind their growing market power? The strength or market power of the RMPs is derived from two forces: (1) market or price factors, and (2) institutional factors. The price factors are more visible and better researched; evidently people save money and time when they visit an RMP (instead of visiting a public health centre) because RMPs are available anywhere and at any time. However, no less important are the 'institutional' factors, mostly arising out of the informal structure of the RMP–people connection, which helps reduce the transaction costs on both sides and adds a strong bond of trust.

The reduction in transaction costs in the parallel market clearly emanates from a mutually beneficial agency relationship, and is hard to analyse by using standard economic theories. For example, rural people with ailments tend to depend on those healthcare providers who are easily accessible, understand their socio-economic constraints, respond quickly and offer a quick remedy at an affordable cost. The benefit of being able to defer payment (i.e. pay for drugs on a credit basis) is a huge incentive to the buyers of services. On the other hand, the providers or the agents (RMPs) find significant market incentives in terms of clients who have no or very poor information about their own health problems or treatment procedures but always look for packaged medicines or injections whenever they fall sick. In addition, easy access to knowledge concerning modern medicines (through medical representatives), good understanding of people's social behaviour and economic constraints, and a very weak public healthcare system make them formidable players in the outpatient market.

The strong market power of the RMPs may be attributed to their efficient adaptive capacity to meet the consumers' needs in a marketized economy. Their strategies are (1) to keep the clinical quality they offer as indistinguishable as possible from that available from the qualified providers by gaining and applying up-to-date knowledge on the most recent drugs, and (2) to exploit social and economic dimensions of their interface to align to their clients' expectations, making this alignment an integral part of quality. The first strategy helps them hide their incompetence (due to lack of formal training) in a market with high asymmetric information and helps make them seemingly on a par with their qualified counterparts, while the second helps them package their services with high client-centred quality elements and make it socially acceptable, especially in poor and backward areas. The formal providers (especially the government doctors) lack the second, and hence often fail to cut into the RMPs' share of the market.

Linkages, responses and impacts

The failure of the government and the formal private market in outpatient care has helped establish a well-lubricated feedback system in the market. The key market actors, especially in a rural outpatient care market, are: (1) RMPs, (2) government providers, (3) private qualified providers (including NGOs), and (4) medical representatives (or drug detailers) who canvass for the chance to supply medicines to anybody who practises modern medicine. The informal (or unofficial) links between the RMPs and medical representatives and government providers are well established. The link with medical representatives is particularly interesting since the RMPs also act as medicine vendors and hence absorb the larger share of pharmaceuticals. Their interface with medical representatives, however, remains indiscernible to a large extent since the RMPs are not officially or legally recognized as medical practitioners. Much the same is true of their links with government doctors, who, admittedly, often 'refer' cases to RMPs and 'receive' cases referred by RMPs at their work stations or at private clinics. The underground link between the RMPs and the formal private providers has also been taking shape; the RMPs often act as the local agents of the urban private clinics or hospitals and regularly supply them with 'patients' for inpatient care on a commission basis (Kanjilal *et al.*, 2010). The mutual feedback system feeds the failure of the above-ground market of outpatient care, consisting of formal or 'qualified' doctors – both government and private. The prominent failure in the above-ground market manifests itself in a high prevalence of imperfect agency relationships, which often result in the use of unnecessary drugs and diagnostic tests. As in many other marketized health economies, the incentive for being an imperfect agent is too high, so that many of these formal actors build an underground nexus with private pharmacies and diagnostic centres on fee-splitting agreements, and make people pay to their advantage. The same incentives make the government doctors engage in private practice, which leads to high absenteeism in public health facilities (Rao, 2005).

How does this situation affect people's health? Recent evidence shows that the rapid spread of the underground market has huge potential to affect rural health (Kanjilal *et al.*, 2010). On the one hand, the RMPs are emerging as 'saviours', especially in relatively under-served areas, since they stand out as the only option for primary care. Also, they seem to possess adequate working knowledge of the symptoms of and treatment for a few specific common diseases. On the other hand, there are serious concerns about the quality of services manifested in three types of RMPs' practising behaviour: (1) indiscriminate use of antibiotics for common diseases and oxytocin for normal deliveries, (2) conducting major surgery without professional support, and (3) gradual penetration of the inpatient care market and specialty care, bypassing the standard regulatory barriers.

Institutional arrangements

Clearly, the liberalization process and the consequent upsurge in the free flow of medical information have created a favourable environment for the informal providers operating in the underground market. Social and political sanctions, coupled with people's trust, have helped them adapt quickly to the changing market environment. At the same time, Indian policy-makers are conspicuously silent on this issue, the possible reason being the inherent dilemma in dealing with these providers. On the one hand, their dominance is too prominent to ignore, while on the other, the legal and technical barriers are too strong for RMPs to be formally acknowledged and their market power redirected in a controlled and guided manner.

Economic theories suggest that a command and prohibitive mechanism is likely to be less successful to regulate the widely dispersed outpatient care market – both formal and informal – especially when there is a high degree of asymmetric information in the market and the monitoring cost is prohibitively high. Legal or administrative prohibition, for example, could hardly check the spread of the underground market since it would be too expensive even to identify the RMPs. Similarly, any coercive policy to control the above-ground (formal) market is likely to make it go underground. For example, the government doctors who run parallel private clinics may still sell their services informally if they are restricted from carrying out private practice. A more effective strategy would be to develop a new set of institutions and adopt a consumer-oriented approach by which civil society organizations, the media and provider organizations were empowered to play more active parts in disclosing and managing information on the activities and results of the health market (Peters and Muraleedharan, 2008).

Pharmaceutical products and services: a derived-growth market

Transition in structure and spread

The pharmaceuticals market in India has demonstrated an unprecedented growth in the post-reform era. The size of the industry, in terms of both bulk drugs and formulations, was estimated at US$18 billion in 2008–2009, making it third globally by volume of production and fourteenth by value (Sakthivel and Nabar, 2010). A recent report indicates that the market is poised to reach tenth position, in terms of value, by 2015, overtaking a few major global leaders such as Brazil, Mexico, South Korea and Turkey.

The structure of the pharmaceuticals market took several interesting turns in the post-reform period. Until the 1980s the market was dominated by the multinational companies (Ramachandran and Rangarao, 1972). However, the scenario significantly changed after the 1980s, and the market became highly fragmented, with the entry of many domestic companies, owing to favourable patent laws and government drug policies. In the post-reform era, with flurries of incentives for domestic pharmaceutical companies (tax holidays, less restricted labour laws, and promotion of special industrial zones in a few states), the market growth continued to be brisk.[4] The market share of multinational companies declined from over 60 per cent in 1970 to about 25 per cent in the early 2000s, and the domestic industry accounted for 70 per cent of active pharmaceutical ingredients and 80 per cent of formulations in India by 1999, making it 'possibly the only developing country in the world that has come this close to achieving so-called self-sufficiency in medicine' (Musungu and Oh, 2006). The scenario again started changing after 2005, when the Agreement on Trade-Related Aspects of Intellectual Property Rights (TRIPS) was finally adopted and India switched from a process to a product patent regime. The market once again handed over the comparative advantage to the big pharmaceutical multinational corporations (PMCs) since under the new regime any drug patented after 1995 would receive patent protection in India as well. The entry of MNCs further fuelled high rates of market growth but, at the same time, initiated a stiff price and non-price war over the high-end products. There has been visible evidence of the market tilting towards oligopolistic competition, since only a few products compete in most of the therapeutic groups (Sakthivel and Nabar, 2010). The market is becoming increasingly attractive to the global pharmaceutical companies as an alliance and outsourcing destination of choice across the value chains.

The strong potential of the Indian companies to emerge as the major player in the global generic drugs market, and a referred offshore location for global MNCs seeking the benefits of lower manufacturing costs, presents a huge opportunity to the market. Soaring costs of research and development (R&D) and administration are persuading drug manufacturers to move more and more of their discovery research and clinical trials activities to the subcontinent or to establish administrative centres there, capitalizing on India's high levels of scientific expertise as well as low wages. The clinical trials market in India is currently sized at approximately US$250 million to US$275 million and is expected to grow at a robust CAGR of 30 per cent over the next few years, almost double the global average.

Apart from a comparative advantage in production, the market has been forcefully driven by demand factors. Increasing dependence on modern medicines, coupled with higher purchasing power of the Indian middle class, has created a solid and expanding consumer base for pharmaceutical products. The rapidly changing epidemiological profile, reflected in a growing burden of non-communicable and chronic diseases, has created a lucrative market opportunity for the industry. The demand for drugs by public healthcare facilities is likely to receive a further boost as the government seeks to expand access to health care.

Linkage, responses and impacts

The pharmaceutical industry has been recognized by the government as a knowledge-based industry and has consistently enjoyed tax concessions for research and development expenses, reduced interest rates for export promotion, and steady reduction in price controls (both tariff and countervailing duties). However, the shining face of the pharmaceutical market ironically overlaps with grave concern about access to medicines, especially for the poor, in the post-TRIPS regime. One reason behind this concern is in the potential threat to India's leading position in the production of generic drugs, propelled by increasing buyouts of leading Indian generic companies by the global drug giants. The economic and public health stakes of losing this position are too high, not only for Indian consumers but also for their counterparts in many other developing countries, as they receive a large amount of low-priced generic drugs from Indian companies.[5]

The transition in this market and the consequent impact on access to medicines is closely linked to the marketization process in the domestic as well as in the international patient care markets. The pharmaceutical industry has established a strong interface with the patient care markets through labyrinthine links of price and non-price incentives. The growth in one market feeds the other through a well-lubricated network of distributors, medical representatives and retail pharmacies. While this has prompted technological innovations in pharmaceutical products and diagnostic equipment, paradoxically it has also strengthened the barriers to access, owing to unhindered increase in drug prices: analysis of price trends shows that drug prices have been outstripping the prices of all commodities since 1993–1994 (Ministry of Health and Family Welfare, 2005, p. 64).

The paradox of increasing supply and an unhindered increase in drug prices may be explained by the standard theories of market failure. On the one hand, asymmetric information propels supplier-induced demand and incentivizes the prescription of branded and irrational drugs. On the other hand, stiff monopolistic competition in the market has led to spurious product differentiation[6] and has helped a few firms control the prices through branding. One consequence of such a branding process is a significant price differential between the generic and the branded forms of a drug (or between generic prices and retail prices); for example, some of the top-brand drugs are sold at eight to fifteen times the price of their generic counterparts (Sengupta *et al.*, 2006).

The transition, therefore, produces a mixed package of social welfare. The innovations and availability of quality drugs have been empowering India to fight dual burdens of disease. On the other hand, uncontrolled prices, especially of high-end products, have made pharmaceutical products a principal cause of economic drain in households affected by health shocks, since more than 70 per cent of out-of-pocket expenses on health care are attributed to medicines and diagnostic tests (NSSO, 2004). The growing concern about economic barriers to access to medicines has caused the state governments to respond in several ways. The most common response has been to increase subsidies on drugs at public health facilities to facilitate free supply of drugs through these facilities. However, the recent evidence from FHS research shows the gross inadequacy of these measures, since a large section of the users of government hospitals are still compelled to purchase medicines from private pharmacies.

Institutional arrangements

The fast transition in the pharmaceutical market in the recent years has cut out an extremely challenging task for Indian policy-makers, especially in the product-patent regime – how to reduce economic constraints and improve access to medicine for all Indians without disturbing the capitalist expansion of the market. Three specific challenges are: (1) how to control prices? (2) how to control irrational prescription and over-prescription of medicines? (3) how to ensure the quality of drugs?

Recent evidence indicates several initiatives taken by the national and state governments, with varying degrees of success and adverse consequences. The policy of gradual phasing out of price control, for example, has actually allowed drug prices to rise at a disproportionately high rate, as mentioned earlier. At present, only 74 drugs, accounting for a quarter of the total drug market in terms of value, are price controlled, compared to 347 drugs in 1979 (Sakthivel and Nabar, 2010). Regarding control of irrational drug use, no significant progress has been made, despite several 'orders' issued by the state governments to government doctors to prescribe generic drugs. The scenario is, apparently, much better for quality improvement. Since 2005, all pharmaceutical units have been mandated to acquire Good Manufacturing Practices (GMPs); however, compliance with GMP standards is not an easy task for the small domestic firms and, given a weak monitoring system, it may even lead to innovations in bypassing the standards.

It is interesting to note that, unlike the inpatient and outpatient care markets, the pharmaceutical market is juxtaposed with a very responsive judiciary and civil institutions. India's transition to the new patent regime stimulated the active involvement of a host of scholars, activists, media and civil society organizations that were highly motivated to raise an unprecedented amount of public debate on the pros and cons of the new regime. The pressure of these players, coupled with political pressure from the leftist political parties, ultimately influenced the government to accommodate unique provisions in the Patents (Amendment) Act 2005 to protect the interest of the generic industry and the consumers.

Civil society groups, such as the Indian Network of People Living with HIV/AIDS, have been making concerted efforts and taking recourse to the judiciary to protect access to cheap (generic) medicines. The judiciary so far has responded positively to such calls for protection of the right of the general public to access those drugs which have significant public health implications (Mueller, 2007).

Conclusion

The Indian healthcare market is at a crossroads. The rapid liberalization process in the Indian economy has imprinted differentiating marks on different parts of the health market. The inpatient care market, dominated by private hospitals, is heading towards a professional and corporatized form of organization, while the outpatient care market is captured by a growing mass of informal providers who are effectively adapting market principles in a poor setting. The pharmaceutical market, on the other hand, not only gains strength from the failures of the two patient care markets but also helps unlock the potential for innovations in service delivery.

The transition logically highlights an important question: what should be the role of the state in such a complex metamorphosis of the curative care market? Should it accept the increasing marginalization of the public sector in curative care and channel its resources to compensate consumers for the welfare loss due to market failure? Or should it contrive to regain its lost position by increasing subsidies and focusing exclusively on better governance in public healthcare facilities? The former option would imply a more active and strategic role of the public sector as a market actor that would provide institutional oversight and social protection, while the second would force the government to play more of the traditional role of a welfare state with reformed governance. The common meeting point for both the options is that the state should switch its role from a passive to an active stewardship role to achieve the following four goals of an inclusive health system: (1) reaching the basic public health goals, (2) improving equity in health care, (3) protecting people from the medical poverty trap, and (4) reorienting the service delivery system to meet emerging challenges from demographic and epidemiological transitions.

The analyses of the Indian health sector presented in this chapter favour an optimal mix of the above two options. Focusing on better governance in public facilities is necessary to safeguard the interests of the vulnerable populations who are likely to be excluded by the private markets, even under strict regulation. This should be complemented with a strategic move towards building a mature social, political and legal set of institutions to regulate the market and offer some protection against adverse consequences of marketization.

Notes

1 This includes three rounds of survey exclusively on morbidity and utilization of medical services in India conducted in 1986–1987 (the forty-second round), 1995–1996 (the fifty-second round) and 2004 (the sixtieth round) by the National Sample Survey Organisation (NSSO).
2 The latest National Health Policy was published in 2002, with a series of goals to be achieved by 2010. Most of them remain unachieved; for example, the actual government expenditure as a percentage of GDP is still much lower than the targeted percentage (2 per cent). Similarly, the targeted basic health outcomes, such as the reduction of the infant mortality rate (IMR) to 30 per 1,000, maternal mortality ratio (MMR) to 100 per 100,000, mortality on account of TB, malaria, and other vector and waterborne diseases by 50 per cent, were nowhere near being met.
3 Some key institutional players are: (1) the Medical Council of India, (2) associations of hospital groups, (3) departments of health of state governments, (4) consumer groups, and (5) a judicial system that allows a consumer to seek justice for medical negligence. There are also a few new players, such as the National Accreditation Board and the Quality Council of India.
4 The financial incentive is compelling: PricewaterhouseCoopers estimates that the cost of setting up and running a new manufacturing facility in India is one-fifth of the cost of doing so in the West (PWC, 2007).
5 For example, 80 per cent of the AIDS medicines Médicins sans Frontières (MSF) uses to treat 160,000 people across the world are generics from India (www.msfaccess.org/content/10-stories-mattered-access-medicines-2010).
6 Which means that a branded product differs from its generic form only in the perception of consumers, not really in content.

References

Berman, P., Ahuja, R. and Bhandari, L. (2010) 'The impoverishing effect of healthcare payments in India: new methodology and findings', *Economic and Political Weekly*, 45 (16): 65–71
Bhandari, L. and Gupta, A. (2010) 'Inputs for health', in A. Mahal, B. Debroy and L. Bhandari (eds) *India Health Report 2010*, Business Standard Books, New Delhi
Bloom, G., Kanjilal, B. and Peters, D. (2008) 'Regulating healthcare markets in China and India', *Health Affairs*, 27 (4): 952–963
Bloom, G.., Standing, H., Lucas, H., Bhuiya, A., Oladepo, O. and Peters, D. (2011) 'Making health markets better for poor people: the case of informal providers', *Health Policy and Planning*, 26 (Suppl. 1): i45–i52
Department of Industrial Policy and Prevention (DIPP), Government of India (2010) Fact Sheet on Foreign Direct Investment. Online, available at: http://dipp.nic.in/English/Publications/FDI_Statistics/2010/india_FDI_April2010.pdf
Future Health Systems (2010) 'Catastrophic health care payment: how much protected are the users of public hospitals?', FHS Working Paper no. 4, Future Health Systems, Indian Institute of Health Management Research, Jaipur
Garg, C. C. and Karan, A. K. (2005) 'Health and Millennium Development Goal 1: reducing out-of-pocket expenditures to reduce income poverty – evidence from India', Working Paper no. 15, Equitap Project, Institute of Health Policy, Colombo

India Brand Equity Foundation (IBEF) (2009) 'Healthcare'. Online, available at: www.ibef. org/artdispview.aspx?art_id=25821&cat_id=119&in=29

India Brand Equity Foundation (IBEF) (2010) 'Healthcare', India Brand Equity Foundation/Ernst & Young, New Delhi. Online: available at: www.ibef.org/download/ Healthcare_270111.pdf

Kanjilal, B., Mondal, S., Samanta, T., Mandal, A. and Singh, S. (2008) 'A parallel health care market: rural medical practitioners in West Bengal, India', Future Health Systems Research Brief 2, Institute of Health Management Research, Jaipur

Kanjilal, B., GuhaMazumdar, P., Mukherjee, M., Mondal, S., Barman, D., Singh, S. and Mandal, A. (2010) *Health Care in the Sundarbans (India): Challenges and Plan for a Better Future*, Indian Institute of Health Management Research, Jaipur

Kumar, R., Jaiswal, V., Tripathi, S., Kumar, A. and Idris, M. Z. (2007) 'Inequity in health care delivery in India: the problem of rural medical practitioners', *Health Care Analysis*, 15 (3): 223–233

Mackintosh, M. (2003) 'Health care commercialisation and the embedding of inequality', draft RUIG/UNRISD Health Project synthesis paper. Online, available at www. unrisd.org/80256B3C005BCCF9/(httpAuxPages)/4023556AA730F778C1256DE5006 49E48/$file/mackinto.pdf

Ministry of Health and Family Welfare (2005) *Report of the National Commission on Macroeconomics and Health*, Government of India, New Delhi

Mueller, J. M. (2007) 'The tiger awakens: the tumultuous transformation of India's patent system and the rise of Indian pharmaceutical innovation', *University of Pittsburgh Law Review*, 68: 491–641

Muraleedharan, V. and Nandraj, S. (2003) 'Private health sector in India: policy challenges and options for partnerships', in A. S. Yazbeck and D. H. Peters (eds) *Health Policy Research in South Asia: Building Capacity for Reform*, World Bank, Washington, DC

Musungu, S. and Oh, C. (2006) *The Use of Flexibilities in TRIPS by Developing Countries: Can They Promote Access to Medicines?*, Study 4C, Commission on Intellectual Property Rights Innovation and Public Health, WHO, Geneva

Narayana, D. (2010) 'Review of the Rashtriya Swasthya Bima Yojana', *Economic and Political Weekly*, 45 (29): 13–18

NSSO (2004) NSS Sixtieth Round (January–June 2004) *Morbidity, Health Care and the Condition of the Aged*, Report no. 507 (60/25.0/1). National Sample Survey Organisation, Ministry of Statistics and Programme Implementation, Government of India

Peters, D. H. and Muraleedharan, V. (2008) 'Regulating India's health services: to what end? What future?', *Social Science and Medicine*, 66 (10): 2133–2144

Peters, D. H., Yazbeck, A. S., Sharma, R. R., Ramana, G. N. V., Pritchett, L. H. and Wagstaff, A. (2002) *Better Health Systems for India's Poor: Findings, Analysis, and Options*, World Bank, Washington, DC

PricewaterhouseCoopers (PRC) (2007) *Healthcare in India: Emerging Market Report 2007*. Online, available at: www.pwc.com/en_GX/gx/healthcare/pdf/emerging-market-report-hc-in-india.pdf

Purohit, B. C. (2001) 'Private initiatives and policy options: recent health system experience in India', *Health Policy and Planning*, 16 (1): 87–97

Qadeer, I. (2000) 'Healthcare systems in transition III. India, Part I. The Indian experience', *Journal of Public Health Medicine*, 22 (1): 25–32

Ramachandran, P. K. and Rangarao, B. V. (1972) 'The pharmaceutical industry in India', *Economic and Political Weekly*, 7 (9): M27–M36

Rao, K. S. (2005) 'Delivery of health services in the public sector', in *Background Papers on Financing and Delivery of Health Care Services in India*, for National Commission on Macroeconomics and Health, Ministry of Health and Family Welfare, Government of India

Sakthivel, S. and Nabar, V. (2010) 'Access to medicines in India: issues, challenges and policy options', in A. Mahal, B. Debroy and L. Bhandari (eds) *India Health Report 2010*, Business Standard Books, New Delhi

Sengupta, A., Joseph, K. R., Modi, S. and Syam, N. (2006) 'Economic constraints to access to essential medicines in India', unpublished report, Society for Economic and Social Studies and Centre for Trade and Development, New Delhi. Online, available at: www.whoindia.org/EN/Section2/Section5/Section446_1683.htm

Shahrawat, R. and Rao, K. D. (2011) 'Insured yet vulnerable: out-of-pocket payments and India's poor', *Health Policy and Planning* (published online 12 April 2011), pp. 1–9

Wilson, C. (2010) 'The commodification of health care in Kerala, south India: science, consumerism, and markets', unpublished doctoral thesis, University of Sussex. Online, available at http://sro.sussex.ac.uk/2371/1/Wilson%2C_Caroline.pdf

3 Lessons from an intervention programme to make informal healthcare providers effective in a rural area of Bangladesh

Mohammad Iqbal, Tania Wahed, Syed Manzoor Ahmed Hanifi, Mohammad Sohel Shomik, Shehrin Shaila Mahmood, Rumesa Rowen Aziz, Zeeshan Rahman and Abbas Bhuiya

Introduction

In Bangladesh, a serious dearth of qualified health workers, in terms of absolute number, skill mix and geographic distribution, as well as absenteeism, limits access to formal healthcare services (Chaudhury and Hammer, 2004; Bangladesh Health Watch, 2008, p. 96). Evidence from an exploratory study in 2007 confirms that, given the constraints faced by the local population due to the inadequacies and deficiencies of the formal sector, the informal sector thrives and fills this void to provide basic and essential health services to the population (Bhuiya, 2009). The term 'informal' includes a great variety of healthcare providers who are unlicensed, and unregulated private providers with limited or no formal or institutionalized training, or without the medical qualification required to provide healthcare services. The informal providers generally offer services from the private sector operating on the fringes of the organized health market. The informal sector includes a large number of village doctors (VDs) practising modern medicine, homoeopathic doctors and traditional healers (Cockcroft *et al.*, 2004, p. 85; Ahmed, 2005). In Bangladesh the dominant type of informal providers are known as village doctors. These work outside a formal or regulated legal framework, and are partially qualified or unqualified non-physician practitioners and vendors of modern (allopathic) medicine. VDs are an integral source of health care, especially in the rural areas (Bhuiya, 2009). Evidence derived from the aforementioned exploratory research in Chakaria sub-district documents that two-thirds of people who had sought care from a healthcare provider had consulted VDs as the first contact, irrespective of the type of ailment (Mahmood *et al.*, 2009). Information gathered from patients during exit interviews was examined to evaluate the treatment practices of the VDs for three common diseases: diarrhoea, pneumonia and the common cold and fever. Evidence revealed that the VDs were providing care of questionable quality, with considerable over-prescription of drugs, and that the choice of drugs was mostly inappropriate and at times quite harmful (Table 3.1 and Figure 3.1).

Table 3.1 Prescription of drugs by village doctors in Chakaria sub-district for treating pneumonia, cold and fever, and diarrhoea, by appropriateness

Type of drug	Pneumonia, N (%)	Cold and fever, N (%)	Diarrhoea, N (%)	Total, N (%)
Drugs prescribed				
Appropriate	11 (40.7%)	17 (15.0%)	8 (14.3%)	36 (18.4%)
Inappropriate and harmful	4 (14.8%)	7 (6.2%)	3 (5.4%)	14 (7.1%)
Inappropriate but not harmful	12 (44.4%)	89 (78.8%)	45 (80.4%)	146 (74.5%)
Total number of drugs prescribed	27	113	56	196
Patients receiving drug treatment				
Total number of cases	9	58	22	89
Total number of patients receiving harmful drugs	4 (44.4%)	6 (10.3%)	3 (13.6%)	
N (total number of exit interviews)				236

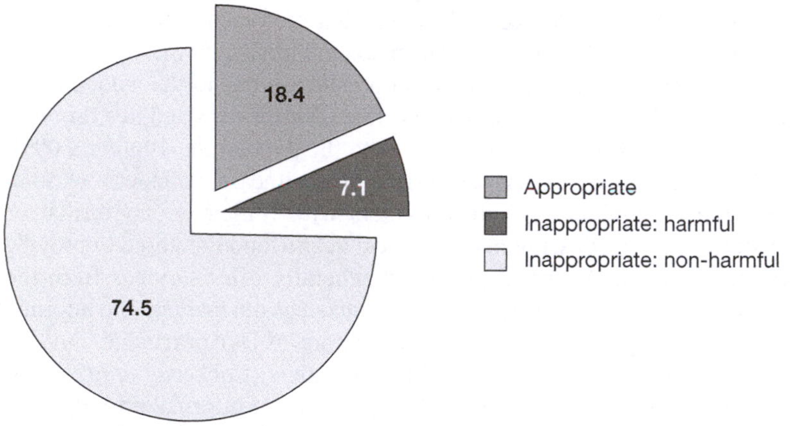

Figure 3.1 Appropriateness of treatment practices by village doctors in Chakaria sub-district.

A review of eighty-nine cases of patients suffering from the common cold and fever, pneumonia or diarrhoea revealed that 18.4 per cent of the drugs prescribed for these conditions were considered to fall within the category of 'appropriate choices of drugs', 7.1 per cent were 'harmful' and 74.5 per cent were 'unnecessary but non-harmful' according to the treatment guidelines of the World Health Organization (WHO), UNICEF and the Government of Bangladesh (Government of Bangladesh *et al.*, 2003). Appropriate use of drugs for pneumonia was defined to include prescription of appropriate antibiotics (e.g. erythromycin, azithromycin, amoxicillin, co-trimoxazole, penicillin). The use of oxygen, saline nasal drops and paracetamol was within recommended guidelines for treatment. However, the guidelines categorized prescribed use of dexamethasone, non-steroidal anti-inflammatory drugs (NSAIDs), prednisolone and pseudoephedrine as unnecessary and harmful for the treatment of pneumonia. According to the guidelines, aceta-minophen and/or paracetamol are the only appropriate choices of drug for patients diagnosed with a common cold and fever, and oral rehydration solution, intra-venous cholera saline and zinc sulphate were the recommended choice of treatment for diarrhoea. The findings indicate that in all cases of pneumonia, diarrhoea or the common cold and fever, appropriate drugs were prescribed in conjunction with drugs classified as inappropriate. Thus, none of the patients was treated in complete compliance with the standard treatment guidelines of the WHO, UNICEF, and the Government of Bangladesh. Thirteen (14.6 per cent) of the eighty-nine patients were prescribed drugs that were categorized as harmful. The excessive number of drugs prescribed for the different ailments indicates that over-prescription of unnecessary and inappropriate drugs was prevalent in the study sample. This study demonstrates a significant lack of compliance by VDs with the standard guidelines for the diseases mentioned.

Table 3.2 provides examples of drugs that were categorized as appropriate, inappropriate and harmful choices for the three different health conditions included in the analysis.

Despite their inadequacies, VDs are a widely consulted and popular source of care among the rural population. The most commonly cited reasons are greater accessibility, local availability, respectful or polite attitude and lack of access to formal healthcare facilities. VDs are also perceived as an inexpensive option in comparison to qualified physicians, as their proximity reduces travel time and costs, and VDs are known to adjust payments according to ability to pay, and prescribe or provide a partial dose of a drug.

Regardless of the detrimental consequences in terms of safety and efficacy of treatment practices of the VDs, attempts to remove them from the health market without adequate and well-functioning alternatives will both fail and deprive

Table 3.2 Examples of drugs in the different categories

Drugs	*Diseases*	*Example of drugs*
Appropriate	Cold and viral fever	Analgesics, acetaminophen
	Pneumonia	Antibiotics, saline nasal drops, analgesics, acetaminophen
	Diarrhoea	Oral rehydration salts (ORS), intravenous saline, zinc sulphate
Inappropriate	Cold and viral fever	Antibiotics
	Pneumonia	Pseudoephedrine nasal drops, cough syrup
	Diarrhoea	Antibiotics
Harmful	Cold and viral fever	Non-steroidal anti-inflammatory drugs (NSAIDs), aspirin, steroids
	Pneumonia	Pseudoephedrine, steroids
	Diarrhoea	Loperamide, steroids

millions of poor people of their most significant source of health care (Bloom *et al.*, 2009). However, the widespread existence of VDs within the rural communities, the fact that they are an integral and significant source of health care in these areas, and their rampant practices of prescribing of inappropriate, and at times harmful, drugs necessitate the establishment of effective regulatory arrangements or appropriate strategies or interventions to improve their performance.

A recent review of interventions for improving the performance of informal providers found that those that focused only on training were unsuccessful (Shah *et al.*, 2010). Successful ones combined interventions to improve knowledge, alter incentives for the providers and establish mechanisms to make providers more accountable for the safety and quality of their services. Goodman *et al.* (2007) reached similar conclusions in their review of interventions to improve malaria-related practices. They found that successful interventions tended to include a comprehensive situation analysis of the legal and market environment, buy-in from medicine sellers, community members and government, use of a combination of approaches, and maintenance of training and supervision.

One way to create mechanisms to increase the accountability of providers is to establish a social franchise. This is a contractual relationship between an organization, *the franchisor* (in most cases a non-governmental organization), and individual operators, *the franchisees*. The franchisees agree to provide selected services according to an overall blueprint devised by the franchisor. By joining the network, the franchisees gain a number of advantages, such as professional training, use of the franchisor brand name, subsidized supplies, support services and access to professional advice (Koehlmoos, 2009). Brand affiliation benefits members by increasing consumer volume and improving their reputation (Montagu, 2002). In return, franchisees must maintain a standard quality of services according to franchisor guidelines; their activities are subjected to monitoring and supervision, and occasionally they pay fixed or profit-share fees (Montagu, 2002; Prata *et al.*, 2005).

This chapter begins by explaining the intervention that was undertaken. It then presents results of the intervention in comparison to results in a control region over the same period. Following this, it analyses reasons for the results, taking into account the comments of three groups of stakeholders: VDs, elected representatives and community members. Finally, it offers some discussion of the results, and suggests directions for further interventions in the future.

The *ShasthyaSena* intervention

In line with the arguments presented in the previous section, the *ShasthyaSena* (SS) intervention, a regulatory strategy with the aim of improving and influencing the performances of VDs, was formulated and enacted in Chakaria. The main purpose of the SS programme was to reduce harmful practices and inappropriate prescription of drugs by VDs. It also aimed to address the poor service quality and lack of accountability of VDs, and establish referral linkages for facilitating better integration of the VDs into the formal healthcare system. The rationale behind the

SS intervention was primarily to influence a large and indigenous group of providers positively through an effective but simple regulatory effort.

The SS intervention was designed and implemented using a combination of three components:

1   improving the knowledge and skills of the partially qualified or unqualified providers through training on appropriate treatment practices and effective use of drugs;
2   increasing accountability of the VDs in the community by involving the local government and leaders in monitoring or overseeing the health care-related activities of the providers;
3   establishing a network of village doctors named *ShasthyaSenas* (Health Soldiers) to ensure established standards of treatment and reduce inappropriate and potentially dangerous use of drugs.

The *ShasthyaSena* intervention had several aims:

•   To create conditions for trust and confidence among healthcare users in the competence and ethics of healthcare providers, and to establish symbiosis between the providers and the users through engagement and mobilization.
•   To create institutional arrangements through the establishment of a formalized cadre of knowledgeable healthcare providers, fostering the provision of responsible, transparent healthcare services by engaging and organizing a group of the existing VDs in the area into a distinct and recognizable entity. The intention was to form a corps of 'Health Soldiers' (*ShasthyaSenas*) who in terms of income, future career prospects, social status and influence would benefit from a reputation for skill and ethical behaviour.
•   To strengthen the local community so that it was able to demand safe, standard and appropriate healthcare services, voicing concerns and inputs regarding provider performance through open-forum discussions with providers and officials.
•   To mobilize local governing officials to show a vested interest in the healthcare system in their locality by regular active participation in open discussions and assessments of the system.

The SS network pilot program was launched in 2008 in nine intervention areas or unions in Chakaria. The project met the criteria of a fractional franchise programme in that the franchisor, the International Centre for Diarrhoeal Disease Research, Bangladesh (ICDDR,B), an international health research institution located in Bangladesh, controlled certain aspects of the network, such as provision of training to members, a referral system in case of emergencies, accreditation of the doctors through branding as *ShasthyaSenas*, and monitoring and supervision of activities. However, it did not control the supply or pricing of the drugs, or the location of treatment. Nor did it provide any other training except for supplying the VDs with a list of acceptable and unacceptable treatments for eleven common illnesses.

ShasthyaSena training

A comprehensive list of healthcare providers practising allopathic medicine in Chakaria was compiled in 2008. Of the 294 VDs, 157 were practising in the Chakaria Health and Demographic Surveillance System (HDSS) area and 137 in the Chakaria non-HDSS area. All VDs practising in the nine intervention areas or unions of the Chakaria HDSS area were invited to become members of the SS network. VDs who volunteered to participate in the intervention to form the SS were required to undergo basic free training. VDs who attended two or more training sessions and could prove their competence by passing the training performance test were branded as *ShasthyaSenas*. Of the 157 VDs who attended a training session, only 117 obtained SS status.

Two qualified physicians from ICDDR,B were involved in training VDs and producing a summary information booklet. This listed appropriate and inappropriate treatments for eleven common diseases and managing referrals of serious cases. It provided information on location, travel to, duration and cost of treatments for serious cases, alongside a telephone directory of contacts. The types of diseases included in the training sessions were pneumonia (including severe and very severe), diarrhoea, hepatitis, malaria, tuberculosis, viral fever, and various complications related to labour and delivery. The treatment guidelines had been prepared in compliance with the standard treatment guidelines of the WHO and UNICEF, and the Integrated Management of Childhood Illnesses (IMCI) guidelines of the Government of Bangladesh. Refresher training was provided every two months, and a phone service to a qualified doctor was set up.

Around twenty training sessions on treatment guidelines were offered to all eligible VDs. Out of the 125 who participated in the initial training, eighty-five qualified in the evaluation and were awarded a crest as well as other benefits of the SS network. The accreditation of peers encouraged those participants who had not qualified to participate seriously in the training programme for re-evaluation. During the second phase of training, an additional thirty-two participants passed the evaluation process. As members of the SS network, qualifying VDs were provided with stickers or badges containing the SS logo. They were allowed to have signboards and visiting cards indicating their membership. Thus, a regulatory arrangement involving a pilot social franchise was established. No membership fees were charged for the certified SS. A memorandum of understanding outlining the responsibilities and objectives of SS was signed between each joining member and the network. The membership was valid for two years. The *ShasthyaSena* members who did not follow the treatment guidelines were considered to be non-compliant.

Marketing the SS logo was the responsibility of both ICDDR,B and the governing committee. After the VDs were trained and qualified for membership, their inclusion in the SS network was announced at the *union parishad* (local administrative level of the government) through open meetings where they received the crest. Through brand affiliation, members were expected to gain beneficial spin-off effects such as increased consumer volume and improved reputation.

To promote accountability of the VDs within the community, a governing committee was established, consisting of thirty-three members representing various groups: the SS, local government, local elites, religious leaders, beneficiaries, civil society, schoolteachers, health experts and ICDDR,B representatives. The committee was responsible for promoting the SS within the community, motivating and supporting its members, preventing misuse of the SS logo, monitoring its activities and providing feedback on performance. SS membership was retained or lost on the basis of reports by the committee, thus promoting accountability.

The ICDDR,B staff conducted focus-group discussions with various stakeholders, and surveys, at different stages of the project. Regular monitoring was carried out in the form of exit interviews among patients.

The intervention was initiated with the expectation that accreditation and training would help the SS members to prescribe appropriate drugs, refrain from prescribing harmful drugs, recognize complicated cases and refer complicated cases to formal healthcare providers. A corollary objective was to reduce the unnecessary costs to rural patients associated with inappropriate prescriptions. The SS programme thereby sought to address the inequities in access to proper healthcare services among the rural poor.

Measuring the impact of the intervention

The SS intervention ended in June 2010 and its impact has been assessed using both quantitative and qualitative approaches. Both the intervention group and the control group were studied. Performances were measured both at the initial phase and in an end-line survey. Data from exit interviews carried out in the initial phase and in the final phase of the intervention were analysed to assess impact on healthcare service provision, performance and trends in practices of the VDs.

Exit interviews were carried out with a random sample of fifty *ShasthyaSenas* from the sample area and a random sample of twenty-eight VDs in the control area. The exit interviews with patients collected information on the type of ailment and symptoms and what medicines were prescribed, along with the dosage and the duration of the prescription. To select the sample, the data collected in the exit interview questionnaires were analysed for three conditions: pneumonia in children below 5 years old, diarrhoea, and the common cold and fever. The choice of conditions was made mainly because there were sufficient respondents available for analysis with these diseases.

The data on prescribed drugs were grouped into four categories: harmful, inappropriate, appropriate, and a category combining appropriate with inappropriate choices of drugs representing treatment practices containing over-prescription of unnecessary drugs. The harmful category comprised any prescription that contained harmful drugs irrespective of whether it was combined with appropriate or inappropriate choices of drugs. The data were then analysed to document the prevalence of appropriate, inappropriate, harmful, and a mixture of appropriate and inappropriate drug choices (as defined above). The results are shown in Figure 3.2 and Table 3.2.

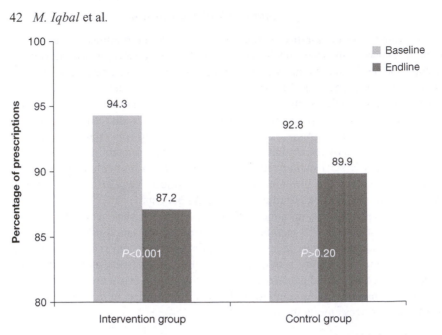

Figure 3.2 Proportion of prescriptions containing inappropriate or harmful drugs in Chakaria sub-district, by category of group and year, including both baseline and final year.

Table 3.3 Appropriateness of prescriptions in Chakaria sub-district in both the intervention group (with SS status) and the control group (non-SS status), comparing initial and final phases of the intervention

Type of prescription	Intervention group		Control group	
	Baseline (2008)	Endline (2010)	Baseline (2008)	Endline (2010)
Appropriate	5.7%	12.8%	7.2%	10.1%
Inappropriate but non-harmful	10.0%	7.8%	11.9%	7.4%
Harmful	13.4%	16.0%	13.8%	24.5%
Mixture of appropriate and inappropriate	70.9%	63.4%	67.1%	58.0%
Total number of prescriptions	491	1,098	167	840

A significant change in the use of appropriate drugs by VDs was observed in the intervention area. Both the intervention area and the comparison area saw increases both in appropriate treatment practices and in the prescription of harmful drugs, alongside declines in inappropriate drug choices. The increase in harmful choices of drugs was smaller for the intervention area than for the comparison area. Further, the combined proportion of prescriptions containing harmful or inappropriate choices of drugs for the selected illnesses decreased from 94.3 per cent to 87.2 per cent in the intervention group in comparison to 89.9 per cent from

92.8 per cent in the control group (Table 3.3, Figure 3.2). However, the results from the difference-in-difference test show that the decline in the proportion of prescriptions containing harmful or inappropriate choices of drugs was not statistically significant.

The increase in the prescription by VDs with SS training of appropriate drugs for the three health conditions is, however, significant. This is encouraging. An increase in appropriate practices was also observed in the comparison group, which might have resulted from spill-over effects. However, the increase in harmful practices in both the areas was not an anticipated consequence of the intervention. The study found that the prescription of inappropriate drugs for an illness by the informal healthcare providers who had received and participated in the intervention as well as those in the control group had decreased.

Analysing the level of impact

To learn about VDs' practice and the reasons why the outcome or impact of the intervention was not as anticipated, in-depth interviews and focus-group discussions (FGDs) were carried out with the VDs, villagers and the members of the local union-level administration committee to help us understand the different dimensions of the local context. The feedback from the interviews and discussions with the different stakeholders provides important insights into the reasons for the increase in non-compliant drug choice and suggests ways to improve the intervention.

In the initial assessment phase of the intervention (in January 2009), a team of sixteen researchers visited Chakaria, the intervention area, to assess the usefulness and relevance of the training sessions. The team separated into four groups. Each group was responsible for collecting information from two unions of the intervention area through in-depth interviews with at least four or five VDs and four or five villagers, and focus-group discussions with the leaders and members of at least two union-level committees. In August 2009, when the SS intervention was well on track, the second phase of assessment was carried out by a team of four researchers specializing in qualitative methodology to evaluate the issues related to the SS intervention. In-depth interviews with fifteen VDs were collected from three unions of the intervention area. In September 2010 a team of four researchers visited three unions within the intervention area of Chakaria to evaluate the impact of the intervention in its final phase. Four FGDs with community members and different stakeholders, and six FGDs with the local-level administrative committee, were undertaken, revealing valuable views on issues related to the intervention. This section examines issues arising from the responses of VDs themselves. It notes their positive attitude, the lack of information concerning drug appropriateness, local demand for inappropriate medicines, difficulties in introducing fees beyond charging for medicines, commissions paid by pharmaceutical companies, and failure to refer complicated cases to public facilities. It examines the views of elected representatives, and then of community members, finding that they largely corroborate the results from VD interviews.

Positive attitude of village doctors

An important factor that influences the outcome of an intervention is the response to, or acceptability of, the intervention within the targeted population. It was evident from the in-depth interviews that the VDs were quite enthusiastic about the training sessions on treatment guidelines for common illnesses. The initiation of the *ShasthyaSenas* in the community was embraced by the VDs as a means of endorsement of their legitimacy as providers of health care. They said that they benefited from the reputation of possessing adequate skills, which fostered trust and confidence in their capabilities to provide safe and effective care. VDs were aware that the level of knowledge with which they provide healthcare services is inadequate and limited in extent. They were keen to learn more about appropriate methods of treating different types of illnesses, and the training programme was expected to be an extremely beneficial opportunity for the VDs. In the words of one VD:

> The people in the community accept me as a doctor and come to me for treatment. With my level of education I would not have been able to get a good job. That is why I decided to become a doctor. Twelve years ago I attended a training given by ICDDR,B. Since then I have been treating people I know. However, I would like to know more and am definitely interested in participating in the training programme. What I do not know now, I can learn from the training programme. I believe my credibility as a doctor will increase.

A positive attitude towards the programme was observed among most VDs, who believed that the community, especially the poor, would benefit through the intervention, which essentially endorses appropriate treatment practices. As mentioned by a VD, 'The people in this community suffer due to the lack of appropriate health care; if we can learn to treat diseases effectively and appropriately, the community will benefit.'

In Bangladesh the state's health regulatory system and the professional providers' association neither recognizes the legitimacy of the VDs nor oversees their performance. As was mentioned by one VD, 'Similar programmes from the government or other NGO sources do not exist for VDs. This programme will help us to establish ourselves as proper caregivers within the community.'

There was a common consensus among the VDs that the training programme is uniquely beneficial for the VDs. From the in-depth interviews with VDs it was obvious that the certificate from ICDDR,B for participation in the training programme was desirable and considered useful for VDs for endorsement as providers of health care. In Bangladesh the informal providers are legally required to have some certification to provide healthcare services in the community and often face harassment by local regulatory authorities. As most VDs practise without any proper certification, it was mentioned that the certificate of participation provided by ICDDR,B would be useful as evidence of training. Interestingly, one VD mentioned the following:

A few days back, the police had come to check whether I had any certification which allows me to provide healthcare services to the community. I was able to show him a certificate for a course I had completed on veterinary health care. However, the next time it might not be so easy and if I can show the certificate [from ICDDR,B] it will help me. I have participated in the training programme but have not been given the examination; as such I do not have the certificate. The patients do not want to see the certificate, the regulatory authorities do. What I learn from the SS training programme will help me to treat patients appropriately and the training certificate can be used for documentation purposes.

However, it was mentioned by VDs that most members of the community are unable to differentiate or assess the type and appropriateness of the qualification of a VD. As reported by one village doctor, 'The villagers do not know what type of qualifications we have as doctors but opt to choose a provider on the basis of the reputation he or she has in the community of providing proper treatment.'

In the second phase of the survey, when the intervention was well under way, as well as in the final phase, some VDs mentioned that training as *ShasthyaSenas* had not given them recognition as para-professionals and that the value of the training was not really understood by the people. It was suggested by VDs that the *ShasthyaSena* concept should be popularized among community members through lobby groups promoting the aspects of safety, reliability and efficacy of *ShasthyaSenas*.

Lack of information about drug appropriateness

One of the major sources of information on new drugs is the agents of drug wholesalers, who visit the VDs of Chakaria on a regular basis. A cross-Bangladesh pilot study conducted by the Johns Hopkins-led research consortium Future Health Systems in collaboration with ICDDR,B revealed that informal healthcare providers consider drug representatives to be their primary source of information on medicines and depend on them not only for drug supply but also for information on uses, contraindications and adverse effects (Rahman *et al.*, 2009). The VDs rely on the information provided by representatives of drug companies on the safety, efficacy and use of drugs. As the drug representatives gain financially from persuading the VDs to prescribe the drugs that they represent, the information they provide on safety and appropriateness or efficacy of use of the drug is generally inaccurate or misconstrued for financial gain. The VDs showed interest in the training programme as an alternative reliable source of information on appropriate and effective drug use. As was mentioned by a VD,

The market is corrupted with many different types of drugs of which many are supplied by bad companies. But how are we to know the good from the bad? The medical representatives usually inform us about the efficacy of the drugs. They advise us about the type of illness for which the medicine can be used and also inform us about the drugs that have higher demand and larger profit margins.

In discussion, the VDs were able to recall some of the practices identified as harmful, such as use of steroids and antihistamine for the treatment of pneumonia. The few appropriate guidelines that they were able to remember were as follows:

* Patients with pneumonia should be referred to proper facilities.
* Medicine is not required to treat jaundice.
* Patients with symptoms of tuberculosis should be advised to have the diagnostic tests done and should refrain from smoking.
* Diarrhoea should be treated with oral rehydration solution (ORS); severe cases should be treated with intravenous saline.

Most VDs were unable to produce the summary reference handbook, although they claimed to have it at home. Despite the repeated training sessions provided on harmful practices and the fact that VDs were able to recall some of the practices identified as harmful, VDs were inclined to prescribe drugs that were categorized as harmful, such as steroids and NSAIDs. It was evident from the interviews that the most common types of drugs prescribed by the village doctors were ranitidine, salbutamol, paracetamol, diclofenac (an NSAID), steroids, and antibiotics such as azithromycin, erythromycin, amoxicillin, ciprofloxacin, cephradine and metronidazole.

Local demand for inappropriate medicines

Most VDs justified the use of certain harmful drugs by mentioning the demand that exists for these drugs among community members. It was suggested that some drugs are perceived to be 'miracle cures' by the people of the community, capable of providing instant relief – for example, steroids for rapid fever reduction, 'What can we do? They ask for the medicine', was the most common answer given to rationalize the provision of these harmful drugs.

> Patients ask for 'Nice' specifically, a drug which provides rapid relief from headaches. The doctors (from ICDDR,B) have mentioned repeatedly that Nice is harmful for patients. But patients want the drug. What can I do when patients ask for the drug specifically? I usually give him the drug he or she requests.

In the village community there are many more examples of inappropriate demand for unnecessary drugs. The VDs disclosed that in rural areas, where a fuller figure is considered attractive, a demand for steroids exists among women who hope they will increase their body weight. 'Most women ask for steroids to become plumper and to look more beautiful. They ask for Decason and Piractin. When they ask for the drug, I usually give them the harmful medicine.'

Another example of inappropriate practice includes the infusions of glucose, saline and vitamin B complex that VDs provide to workers in tobacco fields, who believe that the infusion will help reduce the temperature gain experienced in their work. In addition, a common belief prevails in the villages that vitamin injections are useful in reducing aches and pains.

During interviews with VDs the researchers observed many other examples of inappropriate treatment practices. For example, an infant with fever was prescribed antibiotics (amoxicillin), vitamins and salbutamol even though there were no signs of respiratory distress. Some VDs were apprehensive that if they adhered to guidelines and refused to prescribe drugs that are considered 'miracle cures', the strong competition among VDs would drive them out of the market, as other VDs might provide the preferred drugs. One VD noted, 'When patients come to us, they expect some sort of treatment which has to do with prescribing medicine. If we give advice alone as treatment we will lose our reputation within the community as an effective practitioner.'

A few VDs were not willing to accept that prescribing drugs unnecessarily is harmful. The argument they put forth in favour of prescribing harmful drugs was that 'qualified Bachelor of Medicine and Bachelor of Surgery (MBBS) doctors prescribe these drugs, so how can it be that harmful?' As reiterated by another VD:

> I usually abide by the instructions regarding the dos and don'ts. However, patients are impatient and quite often demand quick recovery. When they have fever they ask for steroids. If I do not comply, they are annoyed and they eventually get it from other providers. So why should I lose my customer?

The perceived effect on patient volume because of adherence to guidelines in terms of not providing harmful drugs was mixed. A few VDs stated that as patients have greater confidence in them as care providers, their refusal to provide the harmful drugs has not affected their patient volume negatively. Indeed, some mentioned that if the harmful effects are explained adequately, villagers usually accept their word and they are able to maintain their practice because of the confidence that people have in them. Other VDs have said that the refusal to provide the steroids has harmed their practice as patients search for alternative sources of care.

In the second and final round of in-depth interviews and FGDs, the majority of the VDs said with confidence that they did not prescribe harmful drugs and that they abided by the treatment guidelines provided in the training. However, they confirmed that some patients were only interested in instant cures and that a demand for harmful drugs existed within the community. It was found that VDs do provide the unnecessary and harmful drugs in order to maintain a stable clientele.

Difficulties in introducing fees beyond charging for drugs

Informal providers and drug sellers should be viewed as people managing a small business on the fringes of the organized sector (Cross and MacGregor, 2010). VDs are generally people who have lived in the community for most of their lives. The close relationship that they share with community members makes it hard for them to ask for fees for the treatment they provide. As VDs are unable to charge for consultations, they tend to make a living from selling medicines, especially those that have higher profit margins. As mentioned by a VD,

> I usually buy all medicine from a pharmacy in Chakaria municipality area. I generally keep a profit margin of 2–3 taka per medicine; for instance I buy each bottle of Moxacil [amoxicillin] for 42 taka and I usually sell it for 45 taka. As a VD, I cannot charge fees for the service I am providing . . . people generally ask for medicine manufactured by reputable companies but also complain if the prices are high.

The existing financial incentives to prescribe unnecessary medicine or over-prescribe certain types of medicine with larger profit margins such as steroids and antibiotics were identified as one of the major reasons for more frequent, as well as inappropriate, use and over-prescription of the drugs. Most VDs said something similar to the following: 'Selling steroids is even more profitable than selling antibiotics. The price I charge for these drugs is more [than], almost double of what it costs. My livelihood depends on the profit I make from selling medicine.' Thus, interventions that impinge on the very means of subsistence of VDs are unlikely to have the desired or intended outcome. It is unlikely that the VDs will follow advice that results in substantial losses of income (Bloom *et al.*, 2009). The priority for these providers is to maintain their market position and their livelihood. So, if they feel that their reputation or market share is at stake or in any way compromised because of a change in their prescribing pattern, they will resist complying with the regulations of the social franchise. However, if they believe that adhering to guidelines will help them to establish themselves as safer or more effective providers in the eyes of the people, they may refrain from prescribing dangerous and unnecessary drugs for the sake of a better reputation and gains from an increased volume of patients. Awareness of dangerous practices and good-quality services within the community may appease the qualms of the VDs about losing their market share. Interventions that intend to improve the performance of VDs should take into account the context within which the VDs act. The financial factor is a significant component affecting the outcome of an intervention and should be included in the design of strategies to reduce harm and improve treatment practices in Bangladesh.

VDs are afraid that charging fees would be considered inappropriate by members of the community and would have a detrimental effect on their image or reputation. As stated by a VD,

> If someone comes to the chamber with 20 taka, he or she would prefer to buy medicine with the money instead of paying the 20 taka as fees to the VD. However, sometimes at night, when we are taken to the homes of the patients, we are able to charge 20–50 taka for the house call.

If I could have charged fees, I could have charged less for the medicine I sell. I have lived in the community for so long that the patients who come to me are all quite well known to me, so how can I ask for payment of fees? People will think badly of me and they are not going to pay me for treating them. They will pay the paramedic who comes from outside the village but will not pay me. What other option do I have than to make a profit from selling medicine?

However, as another VD mentioned,

If we all decide to introduce a fee and fix an amount to charge, we might be able to establish a system of payment for our services, but then each and every one of us has to stick to the decision. If some charge and some do not, then it becomes a problem.

The VDs argued that if, through a common agreement, they could charge for services, then the financial gain from selling harmful drugs would lose its appeal. They emphasized the importance of strengthening the collective influence of SS, reinforcing their 'voice' or bargaining power within the community, and were interested in establishing a local association of VDs (*ShasthyaSenas*) to achieve this. The VDs pointed out that as a group they are better protected from rent-seeking activities of local government authorities as well as from manipulation by medical representatives of pharmaceutical companies.

The VDs mentioned that although their main earnings came from the sale of medicine, the majority of patients were unable to pay for the medicine and in most cases were allowed to defer payment. For instance, a woman who had come to a VD without money was given the required medicine and was told to send her husband with the payment. However, the husband had not come to pay for the medicine.

Commission paid by pharmaceutical companies

An alternative source of income identified by VDs was the commission that pharmaceutical companies provide for prescribing their drugs. As a result, the higher financial incentives provided to VDs by less reputable pharmaceutical companies are a major problem. A VD mentioned that, as an incentive, the pharmaceutical companies sometimes give them as much as 10 per cent of the price of drugs they are able to sell. As was mentioned by a VD, 'Most of the MBBS [Bachelor of Medicine, Bachelor of Surgery] doctors in Chakaria receive about 2,000–5,000 taka [US$22–$50] per month from the pharmaceutical companies.' The companies are also known to have given televisions, refrigerators and other similar incentives to VDs for prescribing their medicine. They are also invited to annual meetings where they receive free gifts.

The people from the [pharmaceutical] company come from Chakaria with the medicine. They give us advice on which medicine to prescribe, which has the most demand and also the most profit. For example, if we sell ranitidine, the profit is high and we are able to sell quite a lot of the medicine.

Failure to refer complicated cases to public facilities

Findings for the interviews confirm that VDs generally do not refer complicated cases to higher public facilities. Whether it is to protect the market share of VDs or because the villagers are actually unable to afford the expenses required for public healthcare facilities cannot be determined from the current research. However, most VDs mentioned lack of financial resources of patients as the main reason why they do not refer patients to public facilities. As was mentioned by a village doctor from Paschim Konakhali, a union where most of the people are poor and landless farmers or agricultural workers,

> Eighty per cent of the patients are poor. The Thana Health Complex (THC) is quite a distance from here. It takes two hours by pull-carts to reach the THC. In addition, the physicians are not available most of the time at the public facilities. Qualified physicians do not practise in this area. So where should I refer patients to? Most of the villagers are landless and poor daily wagers who earn 150 taka per day. The landowners and the rich live in a different area. People are able to get treatment from a VD for approximately 100 taka, but if they had gone to Chakaria for treatment, the approximate expense would have been 500 taka, involving travelling expenses and the cost of the medicine.

However, the accessibility of public facilities is not the same for different areas of Chakaria. In Morongona, a village in Konakhali, approximately eighteen VDs practise side by side in the same area. There are no qualified MBBS doctors in the area. Access to the THC, which is approximately 9 kilometres from the village, is not that difficult as it takes about 20–25 taka to travel to the THC in the pick-up vans (*chaad er gari*) that are readily available.

In the second and final survey the VDs were found to be especially appreciative about the referral linkages that have been established through the *ShasthyaSena* intervention with the formal providers of ICDDR,B through telecommunications. In the second survey, after the intervention was well under way, a group of VDs mentioned that

> the fact that we are able to contact the physicians at ICDDR,B via cell phones is very helpful for the treatment of difficult cases. The easier access to qualified physicians has helped us to provide appropriate treatment, necessary referral linkage and has also increased our reliability as effective providers.

The VDs also supported the establishment of a network linking each VD to a qualified physician. This would enable the VD to contact their appointed physician for advice by telephone instead of requiring patients to travel elsewhere for referral. If the villagers provide fees for the consultation, which should be less than the actual fees and travelling costs incurred, the money could be split between the VD, as intermediary, and the qualified practitioner, as adviser. The financial incentive for VDs to prescribe unnecessary drugs would then be curtailed, thus increasing the chances of appropriate treatment practices. The VDs would still be able retain their business of selling drugs, but only necessary and appropriate medicine would be prescribed.

Some VDs were apprehensive about the involvement of the union committee members in monitoring their treatment practices. However, the majority mentioned that the formation of *ShasthyaSenas* will strengthen their voice collectively and give them necessary bargaining power within the community. As a group they will have the authority to reinforce their rights and establish fees, as well as promote themselves as crucial actors in the healthcare sector.

Views of the elected representatives

The initial phase of FGDs with the union committee (UC) members revealed a consensus that the VDs provide inappropriate, and at times harmful, treatment. They emphasized the need for monitoring the treatment practices of VDs. According to one member, 'We need a monitoring committee in every ward. The committee will watch over VDs and supervise whether they are providing proper treatment, whether they are over-prescribing or prescribing harmful drugs.' The members of the UC did not feel that the added responsibility of monitoring VDs would be too much of a burden, as the community would benefit from the process. They suggested that properly maintained records of treatments by VDs would provide a helpful monitoring tool. However, the UC members felt that they did not have the knowledge to judge the appropriateness of treatment, and hence they should also be made aware of harmful, inappropriate and appropriate treatment practices.

The members suggested that the VDs should be rewarded, for example with bonuses or recognition, for adherence to the treatment guidelines and providing appropriate treatment as a means of encouragement as well as a process of eliminating harmful practices. One UC member noted that 'the rewarding of VDs who adhere to appropriate treatment guidelines will drive away from the market those who are involved in harmful practices'.

The UC members were very supportive of the programme and were extremely willing to participate in the process of developing a conscientious committee that would work vigilantly to increase awareness in the community and ensure a certain standard in treatment practices. The members suggested that the inclusion of influential people such as school and madrasa teachers and imams would be beneficial to the effective dissemination of knowledge of disease conditions and appropriate measures to be taken.

The UC members revealed that VDs are known to sell medicine after its expiry date, which threatens the well-being of the people in the community. In addition, many VDs promote the sale of low-quality drugs because of the financial incentive provided by less reputable or trustworthy pharmaceutical companies. The UC members suggested that direct observation of VDs' treatment practices and regular liaison with the other stakeholders would facilitate effective awareness within the community of harmful practices and monitoring of the VDs. The UC members noted the need to raise awareness of the harmful effects of certain drugs among the community members, especially the uneducated populace.

In the final phase of the intervention, FGDs with the local monitoring committee confirmed that

> the VDs who were not a part of the *ShasthyaSena* network were more inclined to prescribe harmful drugs than the *ShasthyaSenas* themselves. The VDs who are not *ShasthyaSenas* are able to amass a lot of profit from prescribing unnecessary antibiotics, and lower-quality drugs of less reputable pharmaceutical companies. Conversely, we have heard that the *ShasthyaSenas* are unable to earn as much as the other VDs.

However, it was mentioned by the UC members that '[t]here are some *ShasthyaSenas* who by virtue of the training programme have come to know about more drugs and are able to prescribe many more drugs than they did before'. UC members and the other stakeholders believed that monitoring should be strengthened and, if necessary, the power to take legal action against VDs when harmful drugs were prescribed would ensure adherence to guidelines.

The UC members confirmed that demand for instant cures and immediate relief existed in the community; however, 'most rural people are uneducated and do not have the ability to judge the appropriateness of drugs'. One UC member noted that 'when the VDs prescribe inappropriate or harmful drugs, we are unable to reprimand the VDs as they are a part of the community and we have a very close relationship with them'. Another member believed that '[n]one of the interventions will work unless the authorities are involved and regulatory or legal actions are taken when the VDs digress from appropriate practices'.

Views of the community members

From the discussions with the people of the community, it was evident that most villagers felt that they had limited access to qualified physicians. The costs incurred in seeking care from a qualified doctor, especially the travelling expenses, were reported to be substantial. Those belonging to the rural community were aware that the VDs provided inappropriate treatment and over-prescribed from financial motives, and that their treatment was unreliable. However, they sought treatment from the VDs as they were more accessible, and they considered VDs, as community members, to be 'one of them'. The community members are usually not aware of the types of qualifications that the VDs have. One frequent comment was 'We generally seek treatment advice from village doctors who have been recommended by our friends, relatives or neighbours.'

In the final phase of the intervention the FGDs were more informative and provided useful feedback on the impact of the intervention. A member of the community confirmed, 'I believe that VDs have improved a lot through the training programme as they do not prescribe high-powered drugs as frequently as before; after the training they think before they prescribe drugs.' Another member provided positive feedback on the *ShasthyaSenas*:

> When I see the *ShasthyaSena* crest in a VD's chamber I trust them as more competent practitioners as they have gone through a training programme and have earned the crest by qualifying for it and are more able to provide primary care for some diseases.

However, some villagers thought that the training of VDs was a futile attempt, as most VDs continued to prescribe harmful drugs. 'The people in the community have not benefited as the VDs are more inclined to look after their financial gains; they are not interested in serving the community.' One villager mentioned that the extent to which VDs are interested in their financial gains is sometimes disheartening: 'VDs prescribe unnecessary and at times harmful drugs promoted by bad companies for simple diseases but charge as much as it would have cost for drugs of better companies.' Another member of the community said, 'I have seen that ICDDR,B has provided training to a VD and I have also attended an inaugural ceremony of the *ShasthyaSenas*, but in reality I have not seen much change in the practices of the VD.'

The village community believed that in order to ensure adherence to guidelines and refraining from prescribing harmful drugs, the local authority and the regulatory authorities (i.e. the police) should, if necessary, take legal action against those VDs who prescribed inappropriately. They also advocated regulations concerning the types of drugs that should be available to VDs, and would prohibit VDs from stocking prescription drugs that should be dispensed by practitioners with proper accreditation. In the words of one villager, 'Antibiotics and steroids should be dispensed by registered doctors alone.' The community felt strongly about strengthening the Thana Health Complex, Family Welfare Centre and other government facilities at the local level.

The villagers believed that the committee members and local authorities should have more power to regulate the treatment practices of the VDs. In addition, the community should be made more aware of the consequences of harmful drugs, usually prescribed by the VDs, through announcements made at the mosques after Friday prayers as well as discussion sessions held at the community level. The VDs should also be encouraged to provide services with the intent of serving the community.

Discussion

In Chakaria, like most other rural areas of Bangladesh, there are shortages of qualified healthcare providers. The village doctors, therefore, provide an alternative source of health care for people of the community. It was evident that people were aware that the VDs provide care that is not always optimal or appropriate (Sharmin *et al.*, 2009). However, as most rural people are poor, they often experience insurmountable financial constraints to seeking appropriate care. The distance and time needed to travel to public health facilities present additional challenges. In terms of accessibility, VDs are always there around the corner. The medicine that they prescribe is usually tailored to the patients' need as well as the resources available to them. A villager perceives a VD as a provider who understands the limitations of the people in the community, who does not charge any fees and is able to prescribe medicine that is affordable, and if necessary will prescribe partial doses of the medicine needed to accommodate financial constraints. The VDs are also known to be more understanding and their behaviour is much friendlier than that of the formal doctors.

It was concerns about the level of training, type of qualifications, as well as competence of the unregulated informal providers or VDs in providing safe and appropriate health care that initiated the *ShasthyaSena* intervention. The intervention was initiated with high expectations of guaranteeing the provision of safe and effective health care through VDs. However, although the prescriptions of appropriate drugs have increased to some extent in the intervention area, the use of harmful drugs remains a pressing problem.

It was apparent that the dispensing practices of the VDs are driven by self-interested behaviour, mainly for financial gains, as healthcare provision represents the VDs' livelihood. Indeed, it was evident from the interviews and discussions with the different stakeholders that financial incentives are one of the main reasons for poor adherence to treatment guidelines. As persons from the community, the VDs have concerns about charging fees for the services they provide. Ingeniously, they have created an in-built mechanism by which they are able to earn their living through the sale of medicine. Thus, financial incentives exist for over-prescription and inappropriate use of certain drugs. In addition, the informal providers claim that in the community there is a demand for certain drugs that are known to be harmful. As reported by most VDs, the profit or mark-up from the sale of these harmful drugs is quite significant. Thus, training the VDs, who are unable to charge fees for the treatment they provide, and instructing them not to prescribe drugs that have a higher mark-up but long-term harmful effects is probably not going to be a successful endeavour unless the financial context within which the VDs perform is addressed and the earnings of the VDs are ensured.

Most VDs mentioned in the interviews and discussions that demand for harmful drugs is widespread within the community. VDs have argued that patient demand justifies the prescription of harmful drugs. Informal healthcare providers repeatedly inform researchers that the demands of their customers determine their sales practice, but researchers warn that vendors often blame consumers for their own profit-maximizing behaviour (Cross and MacGregor, 2010). However, specific instances were cited where unnecessary or harmful drugs were demanded by the people of the community, because of patients' desire for a quick recovery, and lack of community awareness of the consequences of harmful drugs. It is strongly believed that informational inputs or awareness-raising initiatives in the community can act as corrective measures, redressing erroneous beliefs as well as asymmetries in information between the provider and the consumer. Furthermore, to guarantee competence of VDs in providing safe and appropriate health care it has been suggested by union committee members and the people of the community that accountability of the VDs should be enforced through legal or social mechanisms that aim to regulate their activities. It was suggested that higher authorities from the upazila level as well as local regulatory authorities should be involved in monitoring, and, if necessary, legal action should be taken to ensure appropriate treatment practices.

Research reveals that agents of drug companies represent a significant source of information to VDs on the safety, efficacy and use of drugs. As the drug representatives have financial motives or interests, the information they provide on the safety and appropriateness or the efficacy of use of a particular drug is generally inaccurate. Thus, the strategic design of any intervention should take into account the market mechanisms through which the representatives of drug companies are able to influence or manoeuvre the VDs into prescribing drugs that have a higher profit margin.

Evidence suggests that SS training led to increased referrals for complicated cases through referral linkages established with formal healthcare providers of ICDDR,B. Physicians at ICDDR,B provided consultations over the phone in emergency cases to all SS members. In other words, a network was established whereby the VDs were linked to a qualified physician at ICDDR,B. Instead of travelling to distant places to contact a qualified practitioner, the people in the community contacted the VDs, who in turn got in touch with a qualified physician for advice via telecommunications when necessary. Through this referral linkage, the chances of provision of appropriate treatment increased. The basic role of ICDDR,B was to provide training, motivate VDs to refrain from harmful and inappropriate practices, and act as a referral point, serving the community by providing useful information for complicated cases. It was evident that through this linkage network, the community had greater access to qualified physicians and higher chances of receiving adequate treatment in addition to other factors such as accessibility, behaviour and lower costs. The established referral linkage of the VDs with the formal practitioners of ICDDR,B is a positive outcome of the research and it provides an example of a network that should be explored on a larger scale.

Although the intervention shows some response in appropriate treatment practices, the desired outcome of the intervention to reduce harmful practices has not been fully achieved. However, the social franchise of *ShasthyaSenas* has been instrumental in incorporating the VDs into an institutionalized structure. The training programme has to some extent validated the VDs' skills and has provided them with enhanced livelihood opportunities as *ShasthyaSenas*. This intervention should be improved through research into, and incorporation of, the role of financial incentives.

As a logical corollary of the research, an innovative approach that integrates and engages the informal healthcare providers with the formal providers on a large scale through the use of e-health and mobile technology has been proposed, with the intention of reducing harmful practices and enhancing the provision of quality services, especially to the most vulnerable populations. The suggested integrated system will involve a portal-based operational system that will serve as a platform for coordination of all requirements and activities to promote effective provision of health care. When required, treatment of patients will involve exchange of information, including vital sounds or images of the patients, through tele-consultation between the informal and formal healthcare providers via a secure electronic network. The possibility of effective use of informal healthcare providers as an alternative mode of delivery will be explored in the second phase of the research.

References

Ahmed, S. M. (2005) *Exploring Health-Seeking Behaviour of Disadvantaged Populations in Rural Bangladesh*, Karolinska University Press, Stockholm

Bangladesh Health Watch (2008) *The State of Health in Bangladesh 2007: Health Workforce in Bangladesh: Who Constitutes the Healthcare System?* Bangladesh Health Watch, Dhaka

Bhuiya, A. (ed.) (2009) *Health for the Rural Masses: Insights from Chakaria*, ICDDR,B, Dhaka

Bloom, G., Champion, C., Lucas, H., Peters, D. and Standing, H. (2009) 'Making health markets work better for poor people: improving provider performance', Future Health Systems Working Paper no. 6, Institute of Development Studies, University of Sussex, Brighton

Chaudhury, N. and Hammer, J. (2004) 'Ghost doctors: absenteeism in rural Bangladeshi health facilities', *World Bank Economic Review*, 18 (3): 423–441

Cockcroft, A., Milne, D. and Anderson, N. (2004) *Bangladesh Health and Population Sector Programme 1998–2003: The Third Service Delivery Survey 2003*, CIET Canada and Ministry of Health and Family Welfare, Government of the People's Republic of Bangladesh

Cross, J. and MacGregor, H. N. (2010) 'Knowledge, legitimacy and economic practice in informal markets for medicine: a critical review of research', *Social Science and Medicine*, 71 (9): 1593–1600

Goodman, C., Brieger, W., Unwin, A., Mills, A., Meek, S. and Greer, G. (2007) 'Medicine sellers and malaria treatment in sub-Saharan Africa: what do they do and how can their practice be improved?', *American Journal of Tropical Medicine and Hygiene*, 77 (6): 203–228

Government of Bangladesh, UNICEF and WHO (2003) *Integrated Management of Childhood Illness (IMCI)*, Government of Bangladesh, UNICEF, WHO, Dhaka

Koehlmoos, T. P., Gazi, R., Hossain, S. S. and Zamen, K. (2009) 'The effect of social franchising on access to and quality of health services in low- and middle-income countries', *Cochrane Database of Systematic Reviews*, 1, Art. no.: CD007136. DOI: 10.1002/14651858.CD007136

Mahmood, S., Iqbal, M. and Hanifi, S. (2009) 'Health seeking behaviour', in A. Bhuiya (ed.) *Health for the Rural Masses: Insights from Chakaria*, ICDDR,B, Dhaka

Montagu, D. (2002) 'Franchising of health services in low-income countries', *Health Policy and Planning*, 17 (2): 121–130

Prata, N., Montague, D. and Jefferys, E. (2005) 'Private sector, human resources and health franchising in Africa', *Bulletin of the World Health Organization*, 83 (4): 274–279

Rahman, H., Agarwal, S., Tuddenham, A., Peto, H., Iqbal, M., Bhuiya, A. and Peters, D. (2009) 'Whose prescription is this? Exploring effects of drug detailing on village doctors', unpublished manuscript, Johns Hopkins School of Public Health, Baltimore

Shah, N. M., Brieger, W. R. and Peters, D. H. (2010) 'Can interventions improve health services from informal private providers in low and middle income countries? A comprehensive review of the literature', *Health Policy and Planning*, 26 (4): 275–287

Sharmin, T., Nahar, P. and Choudhury, K. K. (2009) 'Perception of illnesses and healthcare providers', in A. Bhuiya (ed.) *Health for the Rural Masses: Insights from Chakaria*, ICDDR,B, Dhaka

4 Drug detailers and the pharmaceutical market in Bangladesh

M. Hafizur Rahman and Smisha Agarwal

Background

Equitable access to medicine for all is a critical issue in developing countries, where in practice the drug markets often tend to be highly unregulated. The pharmaceutical sector in Bangladesh is one of the most advanced among developing countries. However, with the exponential proliferation of local pharmaceutical companies there are concerns about poor quality of drugs, excessive competition in the market leading to illicit promotional practices and, subsequently, over-prescription of medicines. In rural areas the drug market is even less regulated, disproportionately impacting the health of the poor.

Internationally, it is well established that the pharmaceutical sector spends significant resources on the dissemination of pharmaceutical information by medical representatives (Berndt *et al.*, 1995; Brand and Kumar, 2003; Lal, 2001; Prosser and Walley, 2003). Medical representatives or drug detailers (DDs) are representatives of a pharmaceutical company who seek to promote the sales of drugs manufactured by the company through active dissemination of information about the drugs. Evidence from several developed and developing countries shows that these promotional activities of the DDs greatly influence physicians' prescribing practices (Collier and Iheanacho, 2002; Butt *et al.*, 2005; Akande and Aderibigbe, 2007; McGettigan *et al.*, 2001; Chimonas *et al.*, 2007; Brooks, 2008; Davar, 2008; Ferguson, 2002; Lee *et al.*, 1991; Roy *et al.*, 2007; Tengilimoglu *et al.*, 2004). In order to regulate this sector, the World Health Organization's 'Criteria for Medicinal Drug Promotion' (WHO, 2009) gives guidelines for pharmaceutical promotion, to encourage more rational use of drugs. It defines promotion as 'all informational and persuasive activities by manufacturers and distributors, the effect of which is to induce the prescription, supply, purchase and/or use of medicinal drugs'. However, existing evidence shows that current pharmaceutical promotional practices do not adhere to the prescribed guidelines.

In Bangladesh, as in several developing countries, perverse incentives given to medical providers have been shown to be related to over-prescription of drugs (Adikwu, 1996; Wolffers, 1991; Hardon, 1987), which may cause the poor significant economic loss as well as putting them at risk of antibiotic resistance. An important but often overlooked area in studying the drug supply chain is the role of medical representatives and their potential influence on formal and informal healthcare provider practices in rural markets. The term 'informal provider' is heterogeneous and may include traditional practitioners, unqualified allopathic practitioners such as pharmacists at retail stores, drug vendors and unregistered village doctors. In rural Bangladesh, informal providers disproportionately provide health care to the poor and account for 40–60 per cent of healthcare provision in the country (Ahmed and Hossain, 2007). Limitations in understanding the pharmaceutical supply chain, specifically as it impacts access and affordability of drugs to the poorest of the poor, has restricted employment of effective pro-poor interventions to regulate this sector better.

Identifying areas that can be targeted for intervention to ensure safe and effective delivery of pharmaceuticals to the poor will help shape appropriate policy. In countries like Bangladesh, where national policies and regulations have had limited success owing to poor implementation (Chowdhury *et al.*, 2006a; Islam, 2008), identifying and focusing efforts to engage groups of key stakeholders in this sector remains an area to be further explored. This study presents the available evidence on pharmaceutical markets in Bangladesh and key players affecting delivery of pharmaceuticals to the poor. To fill in the knowledge gaps, the review presents findings characterizing the role of medical representatives from a pilot study conducted by Future Health Systems (FHS) and the International Centre for Diarrhoeal Disease Research, Bangladesh (ICDDR,B).

Objectives of the review

This review proposes a framework to identify and understand the role of key stakeholders, specifically DDs, in ensuring safe and affordable access to pharmaceuticals by the poor in Bangladesh. The specific objectives are:

- to provide an overview of the pharmaceutical sector in Bangladesh and identify key stakeholders;
- to determine national and international laws that govern safe and affordable access to drugs by the poor in Bangladesh;
- to describe the roles and practices of drug detailers in the informal healthcare market in Bangladesh and describe how their practice might affect healthcare provision for the poor.

This review involved a modified systematic review of electronic databases, peer-reviewed literature and grey literature. Titles and abstracts of the research results were screened on the basis of identified objectives for this review. An exploratory study was formulated to address identified knowledge gaps, specifically focusing on the practices of DDs in the informal healthcare market. This study was conducted from December 2008 to January 2009 in nine unions and one township in Chakaria, a rural sub-district of Chittagong district in Bangladesh.

Informal and formal healthcare providers were contacted on the basis of an ICDDR,B-maintained database of healthcare providers in the Chakaria region.

Each of the providers who responded to the phone calls placed by ICDDR,B staff was included in the study sample. DDs were enrolled using a purposive sampling technique that relied on referrals from health providers and other DDs. Mixed methods using a quantitative survey and qualitative focus-group discussions (FGDs) and in-depth interviews (IDIs) were employed, based on a pre-tested questionnaire in Bengali.

Despite a vast amount of literature on interactions between pharmaceutical sector and healthcare providers, remarkably little research describes drug detailing practices and their impact on informal healthcare provision in developing settings. Furthermore, so far little has been done to identify and understand the role of other stakeholders in the drug supply chain. From our research, there is a dearth of published literature to understand the drug supply chain and its impact on the poor in low-income settings. The following sections present an overview of existing published and unpublished literature on the role of various stakeholders in the pharmaceutical sector, and how the interactions between them affect consumers. Knowledge gaps on the specific role of DDs and informal providers in the pharmaceutical market have been addressed by findings from our study in Chakaria.

Background to the pharmaceutical sector in Bangladesh

Bangladesh formulated its National Drug Policy in 1982 (Islam, 1999) on the basis of WHO-specified objectives of access (equitable availability and affordability of essential medicines), quality (the safety and efficacy of all medicines) and rational use (the promotion of therapeutically sound and cost-effective medicines by health professionals and consumers) (WHO, 2009). The formulation of the National Drug Policy and an increased government focus on domestic production of medications led to a rapid expansion in the number of pharmaceutical companies in Bangladesh from 177 in 1982 to over 300 in 2004, and to an increase in pharmaceutical products (Chowdhury *et al.*, 2006b; Islam, 2006). As a least-developed country, Bangladesh is also exempted from the Trade-Related Aspects of Intellectual Property Rights (TRIPS) agreement until 2016, which gives it the opportunity to produce generic versions of drugs locally as well as to expand and strengthen its pharmaceutical sector. Despite the expansion of the sector, measures to regulate adherence to policy guidelines by the pharmaceutical companies and control the quality of the drugs being produced have been only minimally effective. This has led to what has been described as a 'therapeutic jungle' of drugs and drug manufacturers (Chowdhury *et al.*, 2006b). In 2005, Bangladesh reviewed its national drug policy with the objective of improving access to medicines and strengthening adherence to Good Manufacturing Practice (GMP), promoted by the WHO GMP Guidelines (Omer and Cockcroft, 2003).

In the past decade, Bangladesh has significantly improved local drug production, with over 8,000 formulations for the 209 essential drugs listed in the National Drug Policy (Directorate General of Drug Administration). In terms of production, it is now considered to be self-sufficient and also exports about 1.1 per cent of locally produced drugs. Official documents suggest that at least 80 per cent of the population has access to affordable essential drugs (Government of Bangladesh and United Nations, 2005). However, several studies suggest that government healthcare facilities often experience shortage of drugs, and access of drugs by the poor continues to be a challenge (Omer and Cockcroft, 2003; Oxfam, 2006). A number of reasons have been hypothesized for this shortage, including lack of a streamlined supply chain, which hampers access to drugs by the poorest; however, these reasons have not been conclusively supported by objective study.

The specific role of drug detailers in the informal healthcare market

The operational aspects of the pharmaceutical sector, as it relates specifically to the informal healthcare market, can be understood by exploring the role of DDs in this market. The criteria for medicinal drug promotion specified by the WHO proposes certain guidelines for DDs to encourage more ethical promotional practices. Some of the key requirements include appropriate training of DDs, the sharing of complete and unbiased information based on approved scientific evidence with the provider, and restrictions on offering any monetary or other inducements to prescribers. Evidence relating to the promotional practices of drug detailers suggests that they are not keeping to these criteria.

Studies have shown that pharmaceutical companies spend over 50 per cent of their marketing budget on promotion through medical representatives (Berndt *et al.*, 1995; Brand and Kumar, 2003; Lal, 2001; Prosser and Walley, 2003) and inducements ranging from free lunches and 'brand reminders' in developed countries to fans, chairs and other personalized gift items in less regulated settings (Alpert, 2008; Niebyl, 2008; Schramm *et al.*, 2007; Westfall, 2000; Tsai, 2008; Moynihan, 2008). Several studies in both developed and developing countries have shown that promotion of drugs by company representatives influences provider practices (Butt *et al.*, 2005; Akande and Aderibigbe, 2007; Chimonas *et al.*, 2007). There is also evidence to show that the promotional material and information provided by drug representatives to physicians often may be incorrect or inadequate (Lal, 2001; Ziegler *et al.*, 1995; Stryer and Bero, 1996; Norrby, 1996). Various brand reminders such as pens, pads, clocks and other items bearing drug logos are used along with drug samples and other incentives to influence physicians' prescribing practices (Niebyl, 2008; Schramm *et al.*, 2007; Westfall, 2000; Tsai, 2008; Moynihan, 2008). There is a small amount of literature which describes the characteristics and practices of medical representatives who are marketing drugs to informal providers. In these studies, notable characteristics of medical representatives have included youth or a lack of education. A study in Nigeria showed that 89.3 per cent of the 'sales boys' and 'sales girls' (drug representatives) selling drugs to patent medicine vendors (PMVs) were under the age of 21 (Adikwu, 1996). Ferguson found that most sales representatives marketing to private providers in El Salvador had a high school education or less (Ferguson, 2002). A survey in Sri Lanka described how transnational companies have representatives who travel on bicycle or vans, promoting allopathic drugs to traditional village practitioners (Wolffers, 1991). There is some evidence that the marketing practices of medical representatives are more likely to affect adversely the practices of informal providers than those of formal providers (Lee *et al.*, 1991; Barros, 2000). Studies in Pakistan have shown that drug sellers and chemists who commonly recommend medication to patients get their information from medical representatives (Butt *et al.*, 2005). As these providers do not have adequate medical knowledge, they may be easily influenced by the marketing strategies of medical representatives (Ahmed and Hossain, 2007; Applbaum, 2006).

Our pilot study in Chakaria, Bangladesh, reveals a picture somewhat similar to the findings in other developing countries. The research sheds light on the specific role and challenges of drug detailers and the nature of their interactions with health providers, consumers and other stakeholders in rural markets. The key findings include the following (Rahman *et al.*, 2011).

Education and training

Of the forty-three DDs interviewed, 55 per cent had a undergraduate degree and over 40 per cent had a graduate degree. DDs reported that pharmaceutical companies usually require a Bachelor's degree in science or a Master's degree in order to consider a candidate for a DD position.

The amount of training that DDs received after being hired and their reported satisfaction with it varied widely between individuals and between companies. Training ranged from none in the smallest companies, to up to three months of training at some of the more established companies. Refresher training and educational sessions on new drugs ranged from none at smaller companies to one to two training sessions per year at some larger companies. One DD said he had no training, but he felt this was suitable since doctors seldom requested more than superficial information. Other DDs expressed dissatisfaction with the training they received:

> There are ninety DDs in my pharmaceutical company in the Chittagong region. For training, the company brings all of them to one place for a day. Because there are so many people, there isn't enough time to get detailed information about medicines.

All medical representatives (MRs) felt that periodic longer training sessions (e.g. for ten to fifteen days) on medications would be beneficial.

In addition to periodic training sessions, DDs also reported using company literature, pamphlets, the internet and phone calls to their company's product management department in order to learn more about medications.

Income and other incentives

Monthly income reported by DDs ranged widely, but most reported an average salary of 13,000 taka (about US$185). In addition to their base salary, DDs from certain companies received an incremental salary increase based on meeting or exceeding monthly, quarterly or yearly sales targets. One DD stated that if he sold 400,000 taka worth of drugs in a month, he received a 12,000-taka bonus. Some DDs received a daily travel allowance to cover motorbike transportation between doctors. Others reported that vacations to places such as Thailand, China or Malaysia were offered to DDs who, for example, achieved sales of 10 per cent above a target or ranked among the company's top ten medication sellers.

Perceived job responsibilities

On average, each DD visited two to ten formal doctors (i.e. doctors who have an MBBS degree) and about six to twelve informal providers daily. Most DDs perceive their role in the healthcare industry as that of salespeople. Only one DD said that the most important thing was to give appropriate information to doctors and he hoped that this translated itself into good sales. A common function identified by the DDs was to acquaint formal and informal healthcare providers with their company's medications. For some, this included merely naming the medicine and its use; for others, the marketing of medications was required by the company to be more strategic. One DD quoted his company policy: 'Telling is not selling. Selling is a knowledge game.' His company therefore encouraged DDs to provide detailed information about the drugs to doctors.

Interactions with healthcare providers

DDs admitted the use of several persuasive strategies in their interactions with healthcare providers. DDs' primary purpose in interactions with MBBS doctors was to persuade them to prescribe medications. To achieve this, they used informational handouts, free samples, gifts or other promotional materials. For example, one DD stated:

> I normally visit three village doctors and ten MBBS doctors. With MBBS doctors, I give different things at different visits. The first time I will give samples, the second time literature, the third time gifts, and the fourth time I will ask the doctor to prescribe my medicines.

Since informal providers in rural Chakaria often also sell drugs, DDs visited them with the additional purpose of encouraging them to purchase their products. To this end, DDs took medication orders, provided bulk sales discounts and sold medications on credit to the informal providers-cum-pharmacists. In return, for ordering their company's drugs, DDs offered providers incentives such as mobile phones, watches, refrigerators and household furniture items.

In addition to direct interaction between DDs and healthcare providers, pharmaceutical companies organized conferences to disseminate information about new medications to healthcare providers, which were supervised by DDs. A DD from one company described monthly meetings (one to two per area) held by the DD's company to introduce informal providers to the company medications. These gatherings were accompanied by lavish meals and 'mementoes' to help the providers remember the drugs.

Detailing practices of DDs differed for MBBS doctors as compared to informal providers. Most DDs say that MBBS doctors are their first priority for marketing: first, because MBBS doctors see a large number of patients, and second, because the informal providers follow MBBS doctors' prescription practices. Prescription of company medicines by MBBS doctors improves the 'company image'. However, most DDs gave three reasons for spending more time with informal providers than MBBS doctors: first, because there are very few MBBS doctors in the area; second, because informal providers had more time than the MBBS doctors and received DD visits more enthusiastically; and third, because informal providers ask more questions and have less starting knowledge about the medications than MBBS doctors.

Some DDs hesitatingly admitted that when they felt pressure from their company supervisors or managers to perform better, they might exaggerate the benefits and play down the adverse effects of medicines. They exaggerated more often while talking with informal providers because these were less knowledgeable about medicines than MBBS doctors. Most DDs stated that they usually market 'simpler' products, such as paracetamol (acetaminophen), vitamins and drugs for stomach ulcers to informal providers, and the more 'advanced' drugs to MBBS doctors. The more expensive medicines cannot be promoted to informal providers because neither the informal providers nor their patients can afford to buy the higher-priced medications.

Interaction with pharmacists

In Bangladesh, as in other developing countries, pharmacists comprise a major component of the informal healthcare sector and are considered an important source of health care. It is common practice for pharmacists to prescribe drugs to patients, thus acting as informal healthcare providers. Pharmacies play an important role in ensuring rational use of drugs in Bangladesh. Often, though a qualified pharmacist or medical doctor is registered as the owner of the pharmacy, hired untrained attendants or shopkeepers may, with experience, diagnose and suggest drugs to patients. In addition to pharmacists prescribing drugs, several village doctors practising in rural Bangladesh also run their own pharmacies, prescribing and dispensing drugs from their own shop.

In Chakaria, apart from informal providers who stock medicines for sale, there are numerous pharmacy stores that sell medicines, either in small quantities or wholesale to informal providers; therefore, DDs also relied upon these pharmacists to distribute their medications. When new medications become available for marketing, some DDs said that they first target the pharmacist and make sure that their medicines are available at the pharmacy. They then target the local doctors to prescribe those medicines. Regardless of how or when the pharmacist is approached to sell the medication, an additional incentive must often be offered to prevent the pharmacist from altering the prescription written by the doctor. One DD reported that a company's strategy has to be two-pronged: to persuade doctors to prescribe its medicines, and to persuade pharmacists and wholesalers to sell its medications.

Job satisfaction

Many DDs describe tremendous pressure to increase sales, because of the stiff competition between the various pharmaceutical companies. One said, 'It is easy to get a job as a DD but it is difficult to survive.' Another said, 'The competition is extreme: it is much worse than it was just a few years ago; there are so many DDs and so many pharmaceutical companies.' Many complained that their companies set unrealistic sales targets. In order to meet them, the DDs were forced to sell a great deal of medication on credit. When the informal providers defaulted, the DDs often covered the cost of the drugs. One DD said, 'If the doctor does not pay in time, we have to pay the company from our own pockets. We still have good relations with the doctor, cannot spoil relationships with customers.' Other DDs described a perceived change in their social role. Being a DD was once an honourable job, but many DDs now felt less respected in society, saying that informal providers showed them disrespect and made endless demands on them.

Professional associations

Most DDs are members of PHARIA, the Pharmaceutical Representative Association. The membership sign-up fee is 100 taka with a monthly fee of 40 taka. PHARIA 'promotes unity' among DDs and takes action if a DD is being harassed by a chemist or doctors for gifts. In addition, PHARIA organizes informal get-togethers and picnics for the DDs, and supports them in the event of a medical problem. DDs say that PHARIA does not provide any training for them but does provide social support.

Proposed framework for identifying key stakeholders in the drug supply chain

Against this background of the pharmaceutical sector in Bangladesh, based on a review of the included literature and the exploratory study in Chakaria, Bangladesh, we propose a framework (see Figure 4.1) to identify the various players who affect access to drugs for the poor. This framework is a modification of the principles proposed by Elliot *et al.* (2008), also referred to in the introductory chapter of this book. Elliot *et al.* place the relationship between the consumer and providers at the centre, which in this case is formed by the triad of drug detailers, providers and consumers (as identified in Figure 4.1). Evidence from the study in Chakaria helps to explore the dynamics of the interactions, and the influence that is exerted by each of these stakeholders on the others. This relationship is influenced by existing supporting functions, rules and regulation and by the presence of other players in the market.

Our study helped identify some of the stakeholders that impact drug detailing and prescription practices, as well as functions that affect the interactions between the key stakeholders. The key players identified include regulatory bodies, manufacturers, distributors, wholesalers, importers and business associations. It is hypothesized that these parties play an important role in the drug supply chain, affecting not only access to drugs but also the costs, health service quality, afford-ability, transparency, information symmetry and adoption of related legislation.

Evidence from existing literature reviews specific to the drug supply chain in Bangladesh is found to be insufficient to explain adequately the role of each of these stakeholders in determining access to drugs by the poor.

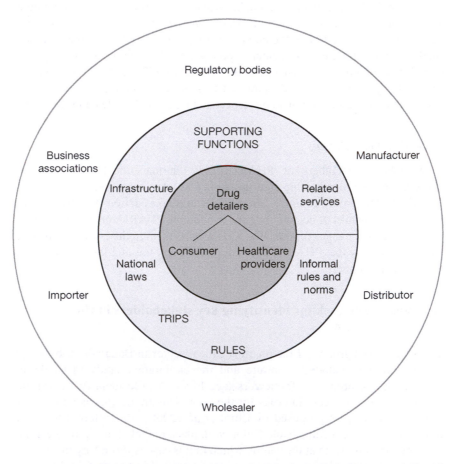

Figure 4.1 Conceptual framework for understanding the drug supply chain in rural health markets.

Steps forward

The conceptual framework identifies the key players and the underlying factors that affect the access to pharmaceuticals by the poor. While our pilot study in Chakaria has made available some information on the role of drug detailers, there has been almost no formal research into the role of wholesalers, importers, distributors and other business associations that might impact safe and affordable access to pharmaceuticals. Our study revealed evidence that associations concerned with health care and the medical representatives' association exist at various levels, providing organizational support and technical assistance as well as offering a platform for discussing current practices and relevant laws that might directly affect such groups. Further research into this can potentially inform innovative methods to improve acceptance of regulations. Engaging the key stakeholders through similar platforms might provide a valuable means to address the provision of safe and affordable drugs at the community level. Our research has identified some of the key players in the pharmaceutical market, including pharmacy attendants, but there has been only limited research on their specific roles. Appropriate training of pharmacy attendants remains a challenging task in Bangladesh despite the fact that this group of healthcare providers needs to be formally recognized to target necessary interventions.

In order to explore potential areas of policy change, this chapter elicits the characteristics and practices of DDs and identifies them as an important medium through which pharmaceutical sector can be better regulated. Pharmaceutical companies need to be incentivized to implement ethical promotional practices. Weak governance may limit the success of regulated policy changes for the pharmaceutical sector. However, a combination of approaches may prove more beneficial. This might include buy-in from large and small pharmaceutical companies and addressing the DDs through their associations such as PHARIA, to emphasize their role in patient care.

DDs are an important resource that can be used as an ally in efforts to improve availability of drug information needed for clinical decision making, especially in remote and resource-poor areas. Anecdotal evidence suggests that similar pharmaceutical promotional practices are followed in most developing countries. Further research in this area might not only have strong implications in terms of furthering ethical promotional practices, but also open up channels to improve drug information networks in rural and resource-poor areas.

Finally, efforts to improve the pharmaceutical market in developing countries have tended to focus on the level of the overall regulatory bodies or on the level of interactions between drug detailers, informal care providers and consumers, the core triad of our proposed conceptual framework. However, challenges remain. At the regulatory level, implementation of proposed changes continues to present difficulties in most resource-poor settings. It has been suggested that the performance of informal providers and drug detailers can be improved through enhanced training and legitimizing the informal providers' roles in primary health care. Consumers should also be educated so that they can play a role in regulating the market for informal providers and drug detailers.

References

Adikwu, M. U. (1996) 'Sales practices of patent medicine sellers in Nigeria', *Health Policy and Planning*, 11 (2): 202–205

Ahmed, S. M. and Hossain, M. A. (2007) 'Knowledge and practice of unqualified and semi-qualified allopathic providers in rural Bangladesh: implications for the HRH problem', *Health Policy*, 84 (2–3): 332–343

Akande, T. M. and Aderibigbe, S. A. (2007) 'Influence of drug promotion on prescribing habits of doctors in a teaching hospital', *African Journal of Medicine and Medical Sciences*, 36: 207–211

Alpert, J. S. (2008) 'Doctors and the drug industry: further thoughts for dealing with potential conflicts of interest?', *American Journal of Medicine*, 121 (4): 253–255

Applbaum, K. (2006) 'Pharmaceutical marketing and the invention of the medical consumer', *PLoS Medicine*, 3 (4): 445

Barros, J. A. (2000) '(Mis)information on drugs: the double standard practiced by pharmaceutical companies', *Cadernos de Saúde Pública*, 16 (2): 421–427

Berndt, E. R., Bui, L., Reiley, D. R. and Urban, G. L. (1995) 'Information, marketing, and pricing in the U.S. antiulcer drug market', *American Economic Review*, 85 (2): 100–105

Brand, R. and Kumar, P. (2003) 'Detailing gets personal', *Pharmaceutical Executive*, 23 (8): 66

Brooks, J. R. (2008) 'Pens, mugs, clocks, notepads and other handouts', *Canadian Medical Association Journal*, 179: 28–29

Butt, Z. A., Gilani, A. H., Nanan, D., Sheikh, A. L. and White, F. (2005) 'Quality of pharmacies in Pakistan: a cross-sectional survey', *International Journal for Quality in Health Care*, 17: 307–313

Chimonas, S., Brennan, T. A. and Rothman, D. J. (2007) 'Physicians and drug representatives: exploring the dynamics of the relationship', *Journal of General Internal Medicine*, 22: 184–190

Chowdhury, F. R., Ahasam, H. A. and Rahman, M. M. (2006a) 'National Drug Policy of Bangladesh: some pitfalls in implementation', *Journal of the College of Physicians and Surgeons*, 16 (5): 368–370

Chowdhury, F. R., Rahman, M. M., Huq, M. F. and Begum, S. (2006b) 'Rationality of drug uses: its Bangladeshi perspectives', *Mymensingh Medical Journal*, 15 (2): 215–219

Collier, J. and Iheanacho, I. (2002) 'The pharmaceutical industry as an informant', *Lancet*, 360 (9343): 1405–1409

Davar, M. (2008) 'Whose pen is being used to write your prescriptions? Nominal gifts, conflicts of interest, and continuing medical education', *Journal of Legal Medicine*, 29: 199–217

Directorate General of Drug Administration, Ministry of Health and Family Welfare, Government of the People's Republic of Bangladesh (2012) Online, available at: http://www.ddabd.org/drug_list.htm

Elliot, D., Gibson, A. and Hitchins, R. (2008) 'Making markets work for the poor: rationale and practice'. *Enterprise Development and Microfinance*, 19 (2): 1–19

Ferguson, R. P. (2002) 'Need for better interactions between physicians and pharmaceutical sales representatives', *Annals of Pharmacotherapy*, 36: 1966–1968

Government of Bangladesh and United Nations (UN) Country Team (2005) Millennium Development Goal (MDG) Progress Report. Online, available at: www.searo.who.int/LinkFiles/MDG_Reports_BangladeshMDG.pdf

Hardon, A. P. (1987) 'The use of modern pharmaceuticals in a Filipino village: doctors' prescription and self medication', *Social Science and Medicine*, 25 (3): 277–292

Islam, M. S. (2006) 'A review on the policy and practices of therapeutic drug uses in Bangladesh', *Calicut Medical Journal*, 4 (4): e2

Islam, M. S. (2008) 'Therapeutic drug use in Bangladesh: policy versus practice', *Indian Journal of Medical Ethics*, 5 (1): 24–25

Islam, N. (1999) 'Bangladesh National Drug Policy: an example for the Third World', *Tropical Doctor*, 29: 78–80

Lal, A. (2001) 'Pharmaceutical drug promotion: how it is being practiced in India?', *Journal of the Association of Physicians of India*, 49: 266–273

Lee, P. R., Lurie, P., Silverman, M. M. and Lydecker, M. (1991) 'Drug promotion and labeling in developing countries: an update', *Journal of Clinical Epidemiology*, 45: 49–55

McGettigan, P., Golden, J., Fryer, J., Chan, R. and Feely, J. (2001) 'Prescribers prefer people: the sources of information used by doctors for prescribing suggest that the medium is more important than the message', *British Journal of Clinical Pharmacology*, 51: 184–189

Moynihan, R. (2008) 'Key opinion leaders: independent experts or drug representatives in disguise?', *British Medical Journal*, 336 (7658): 1402–1403

Niebyl, J. R. (2008) 'The pharmaceutical industry: friend or foe?', *American Journal of Obstetrics and Gynecology*, 198 (4): 435–439

Norrby, S. R. (1996) 'Antibiotic resistance: a self-inflicted problem', *Journal of Internal Medicine*, 239 (5): 373–375

Omer, K. and Cockcroft, A. (2003) 'Bangladesh hospital improvement initiative: follow-up community based users' survey (final report)', CIETeurope. Online, available at: www.ciet.org/_documents/2006227135026.pdf

Oxfam (2006) 'Cut the cost: make vital medicines available for poor people Bangladesh'. Online, available at: www.oxfam.org.uk/what_we_do/issues/health/downloads/bangladesh.pdf

Prosser, H. and Walley, T. (2003) 'Understanding why GPs see pharmaceutical representatives: a qualitative interview study', *British Journal of General Practice*, 53 (489): 305–311

Rahman, M. H., Agarwal, S., Tuddenham, S., Peto, H., Iqbal, M., Bhuiya, A. and Peters, D. H. (2011) 'Whose prescription is this? Exploring effects of drug detailing on village doctors', unpublished

Roy, N., Madhiwalla, N. and Pai, S. A. (2007) 'Drug promotional practices in Mumbai: a qualitative study', *Indian Journal of Medical Ethics*, 4: 57–61

Schramm, J., Andersen, M., Vach, K., Kragstrup, J., Kampmann, J. P. and Sondergaard, J. (2007) 'Promotional methods used by representatives of drug companies: a prospective survey in general practice', *Scandinavian Journal of Primary Health Care*, 25 (2): 93–97

Stryer, D. and Bero, L. (1996) 'Characteristics of materials distributed by drug companies', *Journal of General Internal Medicine*, 11 (10): 575–583

Tengilimoglu. D., Kisa, A., and Ekiyor, A. (2004) 'The pharmaceutical sales rep/physician relationship in Turkey: ethical issues in an international context', *Health Marketing Quarterly*, 22: 21–39

Tsai, H. J. (2008) 'Physician–industry interactions: there is no such thing as a free lunch', *Taiwanese Journal of Obstetrics and Gynecology*, 47 (2): 252–255

Westfall, J. M. (2000) 'Physicians, pharmaceutical representatives, and patients: who really benefits?', *Journal of Family Practice*, 49 (9): 817–819

Wolffers, L. (1991) 'Traditional practitioners and Western pharmaceuticals in Sri Lanka', in S. van der Geest and S. R. Whyte (eds) *The Context of Medicines in Developing Countries: Studies in Pharmaceutical Anthropology*, Het Spinhuis, Amsterdam

World Health Organization (WHO) (2009) Criteria for Medicinal Drug Promotion. Online, available at: http://archives.who.int/tbs/promo/whozip08e.pdf

Ziegler, M. G., Lew, P. and Singer, B. C. (1995) 'The accuracy of drug information from pharmaceutical sales representatives', *Journal of the American Medical Association*, 273 (16): 1296–1298

5 China's rural hospitals in the transition to a market economy

A case study in two peri-urban counties in Guangxi Province

Gerald Bloom, Fang Jing, Fang Lijie, Ren Jing and Wu Huazhang

Introduction

A recent book by North (2005) emphasizes the importance of institutions – the formal and informal rules within which organizations operate – in the development of market economies. He argues that China has created appropriate incentives for key actors in the emerging market economy but that it will need to strengthen its rules-based institutions to support more complex trust-based relationships. This chapter focuses on the health sector, in which trust between actors and the quality of institutional arrangements play important roles. It focuses on three well-performing facilities in two counties of Guangxi Province in China, with the aim of understanding the institutional arrangements within which they are embedded. It shows how these facilities balance the need to fulfil their mission as part of a county public health system and the need to ensure their financial survival in a competitive market for health services (Pei and Bloom, 2011).

China's transition to a market economy has been associated with problems in its rural health services, including rapid rises in the cost of care, scarcities of skilled personnel, quality problems, some weakening of preventive services, and major financial barriers to access to medical care (Eggleston *et al.*, 2008; Wagstaff *et al.*, 2009a). These problems are associated with a heavy reliance on user charges and the incomplete creation of a regulatory framework to replace the previous arrangements to influence health service performance through a combination of political and management control (Wagstaff *et al.*, 2009b). This set of circumstances has created perverse incentives that encourage health workers to rely heavily on diagnostic tests and prescribe expensive drugs.

The problems of the rural health system have been gradually climbing the policy agenda (Wang 2008; Zhang *et al.*, 2009). The government organized national meetings in 1996 and 2001 and issued a number of documents concerning rural health planning, finance and supply-side reforms. The SARS epidemic demonstrated to government leaders the problems that can result from inadequacies in the health system (Liu, 2003). The coming to power of Hu Jintao and the subsequent policy shift in favour of meeting social needs lent urgency to this issue.

In 2009 the government launched a major health reform and committed a very large amount of money to a three-year programme of investment and increases in budgetary allocations for health (CCCPC, 2009). In particular, it announced substantial increases in funding for a rural health insurance scheme. This scheme, to which individuals and local and national governments contribute, largely reimburses a proportion of the cost of inpatient care. It presently covers all rural counties.

This prolonged process of policy development is typical of China's management of transition to a market economy and creation of new institutional arrangements (Lieberthal and Oksenberg, 1988; Bloom, 2011). The government's priority has been to maintain social stability and ensure the primacy of the Communist Party in the face of rapid change. Its strategy has been to define and enforce certain fixed and non-negotiable rules, leave stakeholders a lot of room for innovation outside this boundary and gradually translate newly established institutional relationships into law. China's leaders characterize this process as 'crossing the river by feeling for the stones'. Perhaps this refers to the need to avoid being swept away in the current of change while moving towards a difficult-to-define destination. It is a graphic metaphor for the combination of highly conservative policy processes and radical change, which is neither a top-down imposition of a new framework of enforceable rules, nor a bottom-up construction of new beliefs and institutional realities. It is better viewed as an interaction between a powerful party-state and locally constructed relationships between individuals, institutions and governments.

It is misleading to view transition as simply the establishment of competitive markets. It also involves the creation of institutions to support their good performance. Oi (1999) shows that localities experiencing rapid economic growth tend to have a web of relationships between enterprises and government. These relationships are mediated through both formal rules and informal arrangements. The institutions for a market economy are at an early stage of development, and government treads a fine line in shifting the balance between informal arrange-ments and formal rules (Lubman, 1999). If it enacts laws that do not reflect local realities, people will ignore them, live outside the formal framework and lose respect for rules. If it delays institutionalizing new relationships for too long, the lack of clear rules may generate high transaction costs and lead to sub-optimal outcomes. The political leadership may also have concerns that the expansion of rules-based institutional arrangements could reduce its autonomy.

The creation of new rules of social organization is complicated by the need to reconcile the interests of different localities, age cohorts and employment groups. Zweig (2000) argues that trusted mechanisms to mediate conflicts of interest have become an important element of a strategy for managing change while preserv-ing social stability. Li (2002) argues that 'it is essential for future sustainable development in China to bring about a reasonable order of social stratification with the aid of the legal system'. The government's current priority of building a 'harmonious society' reflects its recognition that rules must achieve sufficient legitimacy among all social groups for new institutional arrangements to perform effectively.

Several characteristics of the health sector may explain why it has experienced particular difficulties in adapting to the transition to a market economy. One is that health systems rely on trust-based arrangements to perform well (Gilson, 2003). People must be confident that service providers will not abuse power derived from the possession of specialized knowledge and skills. They must trust insurance agencies to use resources for the intended purpose. Most successful health systems are embedded in institutional arrangements underpinned by shared behavioural norms. Mackintosh (1999) argues that rules and sanctions are usually comple-mented by implicit agreements between stakeholders, and emphasizes the influ-ence on performance of shared understandings, such as those expressed in the service ethic of health workers. Bloom *et al.* (2008) characterize the combination of formal and informal rules and understandings as a social contract that underpins an effectively functioning health system. The challenge in China for the health sector has been to construct a social contract between key actors appropriate to the realities of a market economy.

A second characteristic is the continued dominance of government-owned facilities and the special difficulties China has experienced in reforming its public sector. Health differs from finance, another service that relies on trust, in this regard (Tsai, 2002). Many arrangements from the command economy are intact in the health sector. Facilities receive government grants for investments and modest subsidies for recurrent costs. They are subject to price regulation and central management of human resources. These regulations distort the pattern of incentives and encourage a dependence on diagnostic tests and expensive pharma-ceuticals. Most of the problems that have emerged are a result not of properties intrinsic to public ownership, but of the particularities of the relationships between different government departments and publicly owned facilities in the present stage of transition.

A third characteristic is the labour-intensive nature of the health sector. The government has faced major challenges in transforming an egalitarian, centrally managed workforce into a labour market with substantial differences in pay (Tomba, 2001). It has managed this cautiously, giving priority to the maintenance of social stability. It has avoided organized pay bargaining, preferring to rely on market mechanisms to determine relative levels of pay between regions and between categories of worker. The legacy of the Cultural Revolution, when many untrained people got jobs, has complicated human resource management in the health sector. Until recently, many health workers in rural health facilities had no college training (Gong *et al.*, 1997). There were strong political and moral grounds for keeping these relatively unproductive personnel in post, putting a financial burden on health facilities and making it difficult for them to pay attractive salaries to skilled personnel. This was a major constraint on health system reform. This problem has diminished as the cohort of unskilled personnel retires and is replaced by graduates of greatly expanded training facilities. It is now much easier for the health sector to establish stable institutional arrangements.

Introduction to the case studies

The data in this chapter come from three main sources. One is the routine management data collected by county governments. A second is a series of in-depth case studies of eight township hospitals (Wu *et al.*, 2005). A third is the findings from a field visit in January 2006 to three of these hospitals in two counties during which hospital staff and political leaders and government officials in the three townships and two counties were interviewed. Although the findings reflect a reality of several years ago, the reforms have not made fundamental changes to the ownership and management of rural health facilities.

China has several tiers of government. It is divided into provinces and then into cities. City governments are responsible for both urban and rural localities. Cities are subdivided into districts. The rural parts of districts are divided into counties and then into townships.

Counties A and B are located within a city near Guangdong Province, which has experienced rapid economic development for over two decades. Local officials predicted that their city would replicate the Guangdong experience. A senior official in a county department of development and reform suggested that enterprises would relocate there from the Pearl River Delta in response to rising salaries. There was an overwhelming atmosphere of optimism among government officials, who projected annual growth rates of 8–10 per cent per capita over the next five years.

The two counties are becoming peri-urban communities. Many adults from County B work in a city, leaving children with grandparents. Many villages have a day nursery. The three study townships exemplify different aspects of urbanization. B1, which is located between its county town and the city centre, hopes to be classified as a small city during the eleventh five-year plan. A1 is located near its county town, whose population is projected to double from 150,000 to 300,000 between 2005 and 2020; a road under construction to the county town will reduce travel time from A1 to half an hour. A2 is a small township on the border between its county and two others. It has dynamic political leaders who have encouraged the rapid development of local enterprises, and it has become a local growth centre. The three townships are not typical of rural China, but reflect the reality of localities caught in the spreading wave of development. Their government officials and managers of health facilities are actively seeking new roles in a rapidly changing environment. These localities are worth studying as sources of institutional innovation that could spread widely.

The three hospitals were described by senior health officials as among the best in their county. They are busy facilities which generate enough revenue to finance their activities. They report high levels of coverage by preventive services. They are clearly thriving in a difficult and competitive environment, although they have incentives to recommend tests and prescribe drugs that generate revenue, like all facilities. Each has a different history and each faces different challenges.

Hospital A1 was established in the 1950s and is ranked by the county health bureau as one of its top two township facilities. It has seventy-five staff and thirty-six beds, and attracts patients from six nearby townships. It was renovated in 2001, the renovation being funded by a government grant and loans. Its institutional culture reflects its long history. For example, it does not have a well-developed and transparent system for determining bonuses. It faces major challenges associated with improved transport to the county town and the rapid expansion of county-level hospital services. Its director complained of losing his best people to county facilities and of an increasing tendency on the part of local people to seek care in town. He anticipated that his hospital would focus increasingly on chronic diseases of the elderly.

Hospital B1 is another long-established facility with eighty staff and eighty-one beds. For a long time it had the best township hospital building and equipment in the county. It now faces strong competition from county and city hospitals. It is competing on the basis of cost and the provision of relatively basic services. However, it hopes to upgrade its services by adding clinical specialties.

Hospital A2 was established in 1989 and has rapidly grown to its present size of sixty-nine staff and sixty-five beds by attracting patients from neighbouring counties. Its director has in his meeting room a picture of a 200-bed hospital and he explained that he plans to achieve this vision within ten years. He visits hospitals and private enterprises in Guangdong to learn advanced techniques and has applied many lessons to the management of his hospital. Hospital A2 has attracted attention at county, city and province levels, where it is known as a 'little tiger'.

The following sections explore the changing relationships between rural hospitals and their institutional context. The first explores the degree to which hospitals can be regarded as autonomous organizations, the second explores government regulation of hospital operation and the third explores the influence of attitudes and expectations of health workers and the public. The aim is to further understanding of the evolution of the institutional framework within which these facilities operate.

How autonomous are these hospitals?

During the transition from collective to household agricultural production, the ownership of the former commune hospitals was transferred to the government. The study city did not follow the national trend of devolving control of township hospitals from county to township governments and subsequently reversing this transfer (Tang and Bloom, 2000). Nonetheless, it is difficult to define which level of government 'owns' these facilities. Township governments own the land, but the physical facilities are owned by the state-owned assets supervision and administration bureau of the county. The county government also employs the hospital director and other permanent employees, sets performance targets and monitors their achievement.

Hospital managers have a lot of autonomy over financial decisions. Government provides investment finance and minimal levels of support for recurrent expenditure. The hospitals finance over 90 per cent of their annual expenditure on salaries and their own investment in training, equipment and buildings. Hospital directors lobby for government investment, but they also borrow money to finance improvements. The finance department of the county health bureaux reported that its staff had little information about the level of borrowing, and there is every indication that hospitals have a lot of freedom. On the other hand, some command economy regulations continue to constrain management autonomy, such as the control of prices and human resources.

It is difficult to characterize these facilities as public or private. They use surpluses to pay salary bonuses or invest. They are subject to a number of regulations and government targets, but there is scope for entrepreneurship. It is also difficult to define the relative importance of different stakeholders in hospital decisions. Permanent employees have significant influence. The hospitals have elaborate systems to ensure rules-based allocation of surpluses, particularly for salary bonuses. But government has little reliable information about hospital finances.

Regulation: creating the institutions of a socially responsible market

A number of studies have documented the financial incentives that encourage health facilities to provide costly care that depends on diagnostic tests and a high volume of drug prescriptions (Eggleston *et al.*, 2008; Wagstaff *et al.*, 2009a). These arise from their heavy reliance on patients' payments and the controlled prices, which do not cover the cost of medical consultations but permit health facilities to earn profits from selling drugs and using medical equipment. All payment systems create incentives that can lead to deleterious outcomes if there are no countervailing influences. This section explores how the study counties have tried to create such countervailing influences through formal rules and informal arrangements.

China is governed by four sets of leadership bodies replicated at every administrative level: the Communist Party, the Government Administration, the People's Congress and the People's Political Consultative Conference. The Chinese Constitution defines a leading role for the Communist Party. The Party leads policy debates and controls the appointment of government officials and reviews their performance annually. This review strongly influences their promotion prospects (Huang, 1995). The rise of health on the policy agenda has meant that health is taken into account in these assessments. The Communist Party is present at all workplaces, and the local Party Secretary influences decisions. The Party also acts as a network through which hospitals seek assistance in meeting their objectives.

The government is organized into a number of departments. At each administrative level the department is answerable to the local government, but is strongly influenced by national policies and guidelines. Departments relevant to rural hospitals include health, planning and reform, finance, price, civil affairs, food and drug supervision, and human resources. Their roles are discussed in what follows. There are no formal arrangements to coordinate health-related functions.

Two bodies supervise government operation. The People's Congress oversees and supervises government administration and the civil and criminal courts. This is called supervision over the 'one government and two courts' (*yifu liang yuan*). It meets annually, and standing committees respond more frequently to problems and complaints. The People's Political Consultative Conference performs 'democratic supervision' over government administration. It holds an annual conference and its standing committees hold irregular meetings. According to the Deputy Director of the Political Consultative Conference of County B, its 'democratic supervision' is less powerful than 'legal supervision' by the People's Congress.

The county health bureau is formally responsible for the performance of township hospitals. It appoints their directors, subject to approval by the Communist Party, and signs a three-year contract with the director, which defines the hospital's mission and sets performance targets. Hospitals are required to make a small deposit at the beginning of the year, to be refunded if they perform well. A team of eight to ten people from the county health bureau makes two monitoring visits a year to each hospital. Good performers have their deposits reimbursed and are praised at meetings for hospital directors. The financial incentives are small, but being graded as good or bad is taken seriously. The health bureaux have other powers. They influence the allocation of government grants for recurrent expenditure and the investment funds from higher levels of government. They also carry out annual reviews of hospital directors, influence the allocation of skilled staff between health facilities and approve proposals to invest in major equipment and improvements in buildings. Hospital directors have good reasons to take monitoring visits seriously.

One sign of health bureau influence is the high level of coverage by preventive programmes, despite minimal government funding. The three hospitals have dynamic preventive departments, which organize immunization and maternal health care. Several factors contribute to this outcome. First is the publication of clear coverage targets. Second is government funding for centres for disease control and maternal and child health, linked with mandates to monitor achievement of targets. These centres ensure that the targets are included in the contracts with the hospital directors, provide technical support and monitor performance. The County B Centre for Disease Control carries out small surveys to validate reported coverage. Finally, the county and provincial health departments have made it clear that they take preventive programmes seriously. The hospital directors complained of the financial burden these programmes placed on their facility and hoped that government would eventually finance essential public health services. Meanwhile, they continue to take them seriously, despite the financial disincentives.

Another factor that may have encouraged hospitals to support maternal health services is the advantage that government regulations have given them. Counties A and B made it illegal for village midwives to carry out home deliveries several years ago, although the practice continues in the more remote villages. Some township governments only register births that take place in a facility based in the county. These actions have been associated with rapid increases in demand for hospital-based obstetric care. The obstetrics department has become the busiest in Hospital B1. This may explain why hospitals actively support community-based maternal health services and are willing to pay 30–50 yuan per patient to village midwives for undertaking antenatal examinations and making referrals to hospital. This illustrates the regulatory partnership developing between government and public hospitals.

This partnership is viable largely because of growing demand linked to rising household incomes due to the increasing availability of work in urban areas. It is also likely that attitudes towards health care are changing and that people are more actively seeking preventive services and what they perceive to be 'modern' hospital deliveries.

The government has been less successful in promoting cost-effective medical treatment. It continues to exercise powers from the command economy period. Those important to rural hospitals concern human resources, investments and prices. The human resources department approves all appointments to permanent posts. Some time ago, rural health facilities became increasingly overstaffed, in part as a result of inappropriate use of government powers. This situation seems to have changed in the study counties, where the current aim is to control staff numbers, reflecting central government's support for personnel reform. County A has frozen the number of permanent posts in the health sector, and most recruitment is on the basis of fixed-term contracts. According to hospital directors, this has limited their ability to attract the best candidates. All directors attend fairs at which new graduates seek jobs. They reported that new graduates of medical schools are increasingly interested in jobs in township hospitals. This is a major change in the medical labour market, resulting from an expansion in health worker training.

The county health bureau reviews plans to purchase large pieces of equipment and invest in buildings. The hospital directors said that it is not difficult to gain approval for self-financed investments. The county health bureau also influences the allocation of investment funding from higher levels of government. These decisions have been made without a formal health resource plan. There is a general air of optimism among managers of county-level facilities, who expect that growth in the urban population, rising incomes and anticipated increases in government health expenditure will lead to large increases in demand. These facilities have already expanded their services and purchased major equipment, such as computerized tomography (CT) scanners, or they intend to do so. The lack of an agreed plan or of a management body with overall responsibility for the health system has made it difficult for relatively small township facilities to anticipate their niche in a rapidly changing health system. The study city is presently producing its first regional health plan.

The price bureau sets prices for health goods and services. A long-established strategy for ensuring affordability has been to keep charges for professional consultations and inpatient beds low, and permit health facilities to earn money by charging for pharmaceuticals and tests. However, there is much discontent about the high costs of medical care. In late 2005 the Guangxi Provincial Price Bureau reduced charges for tests and a number of drugs. The directors of the township hospitals expressed concern that this change would create serious difficulties. In practice, hospitals do not always adhere to the official price schedule. The county price bureau carries out routine visits to health facilities and responds to complaints about overcharging. The most common punishment is to require the hospital to refund clients and/or pay a fine. The relevant officials said they kept fines low because of the financial difficulties of the hospitals. They also said that local officials or political leaders sometimes pressured them to be lenient. This illustrates how regulators balance competing objectives of keeping medical costs low and enabling health facilities to finance their activities. The price bureaux in the two counties did not have to meet quotas for collecting fines and they had adequate budgets to carry out their duties. Their situation is different from that of a poor county in Guizhou Province, where a recent study found the enforcement of price controls had a strong rent-seeking element.

The increasing importance of market relationships has created new challenges for government. A senior provincial official outlined a typology of competition. Competition between employees of health facilities, he said, is an appropriate response to the need to attract patients. Competition between facilities is either orderly or disorderly. The latter is against the interest of the community, and government has to protect people against sub-standard or dangerous practices. This provided his rationale for the design of a regulatory framework.

The government sets minimum standards for health service providers. All small hospitals have to apply for a licence from the city government and are inspected every three years. Village doctors must pass an annual licensing examination. County B recently prohibited village clinics from providing intravenous treatment. This is an important measure to protect the public against unnecessary costs and risks. The government has also introduced laws to control the right to prescribe certain drugs. In addition to protecting the public, these regulations shield township hospitals from competition.

The government has created a Food and Drug Regulatory Agency (FDRA) to reduce the risk from ineffective or dangerous pharmaceuticals. The FDRAs in the study counties were established in 2002. They are actually answerable to the city government, which shields them from pressure by county and township governments to soften enforcement. The two county agencies have enough funding to visit facilities regularly. Their major task is to ensure that hospitals and drugstores procure pharmaceuticals from suppliers that meet minimum quality standards. Suppliers must provide purchasers with a copy of their operating licence. Hospitals and drugstores can be fined if they buy drugs from unregulated sources. All drugstores are required to obtain a licence. Since 2003 the government has differentiated between over-the-counter drugs and those for which a prescription is required, although the study counties have not begun to enforce this regulation.

The officials of the two county FDRAs said that their major emphasis was on altering understandings of the risks of low-quality drugs and the responsibilities of health service providers. One important innovation has been the establishment of voluntary associations in both counties. The Pharmaceutical Association of County B has 95 per cent of all drugstores as members. Members pay an annual fee that depends on the kind of facility, beginning with 200 yuan for village ones. They promise to supply only legal drugs and are entitled to display a certificate in their premise. They are also expected to report illegally supplied products. The association has independent legal status and is registered with the Department of Civil Affairs. Its director is the deputy director of the county FDRA. It is difficult to say whether membership is truly voluntary and members derive benefits from displaying their membership certificate. However, the decision to create it suggests that government believes it needs the active support of public and private facilities and pharmacies to regulate drugs effectively. It is difficult to predict the degree to which the association will eventually act as an independent stakeholder in the county health system.

All societies have mechanisms to ensure that people with specialized skills and knowledge do not abuse their powers. These commonly combine a service ethic with measures to control opportunistic behaviour. Many societies establish self-regulating professions to influence health worker behaviour. China has chosen not to create this kind of independent body. It encourages ethical behaviour through political exhortation and control. The Communist Party has established Disciplinary Inspection Committees (DICs) to monitor the integrity of leaders of different government departments and prevent corruption. In the early 1990s it established the Rectifying Incorrect Professional Ethics Office (RIPEO) within these committees to counteract bad behaviour by public service departments (Fang, 2008).

The decision by the two county RIPEOs to focus on health followed the 1996 national meeting, described above, at which policy-makers acknowledged that rural health services had serious problems. The County A RIPEO launched a campaign to improve practices in the health sector in 1998. According to RIPEO officials, there is a clear distinction between professional competence, which is the health bureau's concern, and unethical behaviour, for which they are responsible. They have focused on procurement for construction projects, management of pharmaceuticals and informal payments, known as 'red packages'.

The RIPEOs undertake a number of activities. Every county health facility must appoint a supervisor of professional ethics, and the director plays this role in township hospitals. Each hospital submits an annual ethics report. The RIPEO carries out educational activities for hospital staff. It runs a complaint hotline and undertakes opinion polls on health system performance. According to RIPEO staff, there has been a marked decrease in the number of complaints about unethical behaviour. The city government has honoured County B County Hospital by selecting it as the venue for a city-wide conference on the creation of a service culture.

The People's Congress also monitors bad behaviour. People can express their views through letters or telephone calls. It reviews health bureau performance annually. It also carries out regular supervision visits of health facilities with representatives of the price bureau, audit and other supervisory units. If it finds wrongdoing, it orders the hospitals to correct it and informs relevant government departments.

Township hospitals in the two counties operate within a web of relationships aimed at ensuring they take the community's interest into account. These arrangements have influenced facilities to achieve good coverage by preventive programmes. They have been less successful in controlling medical care costs. The government has created parallel institutions to monitor provider performance, with limited effect. Openly unethical behaviour, such as accepting kickbacks from suppliers and demanding red packages, has diminished since the late 1990s. However, complaints about prices have continued, and cost is a significant barrier to access to medical care. The decision by the Guangxi government to reduce prices in late 2005 was one more attempt to address this problem with bureaucratic measures.

Building trust

A common thread running through many discussions with officials of the county RIPEOs, FDRAs, People's Congress and People's Political Consultative Congress was the need to increase the public's trust in the health system. Interviewees emphasized the need to change attitudes and discourage opportunistic behaviour. One senior official discussed this issue in depth. He had overseen a major effort to eliminate kickbacks and requests for red packages. Several people were fired and some township hospital directors were disciplined. He is now concerned to ensure that the new rural health insurance scheme, known as the New Cooperative Medical System (NCMS), will succeed. Several years ago a government agricultural credit agency collapsed, leaving many people out of pocket. This collapse damaged trust, and the county government has to convince people that higher levels of government will not suddenly withdraw support from the NCMS and that the funds will be used appropriately. He saw this as the greatest hurdle to be overcome.

The hospital directors were also concerned with building trust. This was a strong theme in Township B2, where the hospital has made great efforts to strengthen its relationship with the community. Its director meets patients and their families every three months to discuss their experiences and identify problems. He organizes an annual sporting week during which the community is encouraged to watch games in the hospital grounds. He sees these activities as part of an effort to build links between the community and the hospital. Other hospital directors are less active, but they all describe work on preventive programmes as a way to create new relationships with potential patients.

One reason for the interest in the hospital's reputation is the competition for patients between township hospitals, village doctors and county- and city-level hospitals. Most households have a family member working in a city. They are experiencing rises in income. This, combined with the increasing number of trained village doctors and greatly improved transport, has meant that people have a much greater choice of providers. They also have access to many more sources of information and their expectations have changed. One hospital doctor said that they had to upgrade their medical equipment to keep up with facilities in Guangdong Province, where many local people worked. For example, people would only trust laboratory tests if the results were printed by a computer. All three hospital directors tried to attract patients by upgrading services and keeping costs down. They found it difficult to achieve this and still pay their employees competitive salaries.

The most important government strategy for managing conflicts of interest between providers and the public is through the systems for supervising performance, described in the previous section. The government has opened channels for people to express their dissatisfaction. Each hospital puts the names and pictures of staff on the wall and provides a telephone number for complaints. It also provides a box for written complaints. The hospitals said that they receive very few complaints. Officials of the People's Congress and the People's Political Consultative Conference also said they receive few health-related complaints. People seem more willing to change provider than exercise their voice, except when a major problem arises. The director of County A Health Bureau said that his most difficult task was dealing with the aftermath of deaths. On two occasions in 2005, many villagers occupied a township hospital after a death, demanding compensation. He had to spend a lot of time and energy to resolve these disputes.

In 2003 the government announced a major initiative as part of a broader policy shift in favour of the rural poor. It launched the already mentioned new rural health insurance scheme, known as the NCMS, with the stated aim of reducing the risk of household impoverishment due to a major illness. At first, the central government allocated 10 yuan per person covered by a scheme, as long as contributions by local governments and household contributions each matched it. Both levels of government have subsequently increased their contributions. The schemes use most of their funds to reimburse a proportion of the cost of hospital care. County B was one of the initial 300 pilot counties, and County A is establishing its scheme.

Discussions in County B suggest that the NCMS is seen by government officials as an important initiative. Several people said that the NCMS and the abolition of the agricultural tax were the most visible manifestations of the government's concern for the rural poor. Local government leaders appear to have a strong stake in its success. The County B NCMS is organized by the county health bureau. The government's main aim has been to establish the scheme quickly and build trust in its financial management. The scheme produces detailed accounts. It established a supervisory committee that includes representatives of the price bureau, auditing bureau, civil affairs bureau, the Discipline Inspection Committee of the Communist Party, the People's Political Consultative Conference and the People's Congress. This committee has focused on ensuring that money was used for the appropriate purpose and that reimbursement was transparent.

It is too early to assess the impact of the NCMS on health system performance. Experiences with previous schemes revealed problems with rises in medical costs and disproportionate access to benefits by the better-off and those living near large hospitals. The county has not paid attention to these issues yet. However, the scheme is establishing a computerized information system that will provide detailed information on the treatment of each case and will make it possible to assess the distribution of benefits among the population. Depending on how this information is used, the NCMS could provide an institutional basis for the negotiation of new trust-based arrangements in the rural health sector.

Conclusions

The findings in the two counties illustrate the web of relationships within which township hospitals operate. These arrangements emerged during the early years of transition to a market economy, when government's priority was to prevent social disorder while individuals and institutions adapted to radical changes in the economic system. The options were limited by, among other things, the absence of a labour market, scarcities of trained health workers and weaknesses in local government management and governance. The government's strategy was to guarantee basic salaries, keep prices of essential services low and encourage enterprises (including hospitals) to generate revenue (Bloom, 2005). This resulted in rapid economic growth, and most health facilities avoided financial collapse. However, the slowness in replacing previous values and institutional arrangements for constraining unacceptable behaviour with new ones discouraged the development of trust-based relationships. Hospitals' strategies for avoiding bankruptcy contributed to a widespread perception that they put their own interests above those of patients. This contributed to a decay of trust.

The government has responded in several ways. First, it has used its financial resources and regulatory powers to induce health facilities to provide benefits to the population. This has worked well with preventive programmes, where targets have been clearly defined, specific institutions have been made responsible for ensuring that targets are met and the cost to hospitals of achieving defined objectives is not great. It has worked much less well in ensuring that care is appropriate and affordable. Hospitals have found it difficult to reconcile the achievement of this objective with their need to generate revenue. Government regulatory agencies have recognized these conflicting objectives and they have tried to avoid measures that could jeopardize the financial viability of hospitals. Also, the targets are less clearly defined and no single agency is responsible for monitoring their achievement.

It is important to keep in mind that the hospitals studied are among the most successful in the two counties. They generate enough revenue from paying patients to subsidize preventive services. They also take a relatively long-term view of the value of building their reputation. These considerations apply much less to facilities in poorer localities or with low-quality staff, where the main concern is day-to-day financial survival, and preventive services may be much weaker. The present approach has fostered the emergence of very great differences between the best- and worst-served localities.

Second, it has restructured relationships between government departments to alter the balance of influences on providers. The Health Department of each level of government is perceived to represent its own facilities and personnel. This is one reason why government assigned management of urban health insurance to the Ministry of Labour and Social Security. It has not replicated this pattern in the rural health services, leaving management of the NCMS to county health bureaux. But it has required schemes to establish supervisory bodies on which all sectors are represented. These supervisory bodies have focused mostly on financial transparency, but they could eventually provide a counterbalance to the interests of providers. The government has also given control over the use of funds allocated for its new health safety net to the Ministry of Civil Affairs. Another institutional innovation has been to make county-level departments of the FDRA directly answerable to the city government, thereby reducing the influence of local stakeholders on enforcement. The balancing of institutional interests in these arrangements appears to have helped reduce bad behaviour. However, many problems persist.

Third, it has defined more clearly the boundary between acceptable and unacceptable behaviour and fostered changes in understandings of ethical behaviour. Doing so has been the responsibility of specialized regulatory agencies and of the RIPEO of the Communist Party, which labels certain activities as 'corrupt' and disciplines transgressors. As government has widened the regulatory framework, with rules to ensure drug quality and safety or to license village doctors, for example, additional behaviours have been labelled corrupt and/or illegal. The definition of unacceptable behaviour has gradually widened. Both the RIPEO and the regulatory agencies, such as the FDRA, refer to the need to alter attitudes and create expectations that providers both 'will' and 'ought to' follow new behavioural norms. They organize educational activities to achieve this. They argue that new norms of professional behaviour are gradually being established. They do not comment on the impact on public expectations.

The experiences of the two counties illustrate the importance of government commitment to the performance of the health sector. The effort of the RIPEOs has been a response to the growing government concern about the performance of health providers. The success of the preventive programmes, the gradual development of a regulatory framework and the establishment of NCMS are all part of this response. One gets a sense of a growing consensus around what constitutes appropriate behaviour by rural hospitals. All three hospital directors gave the impression that their facility had to be seen to perform well for their facility to benefit from government resource allocation and use of regulatory powers. They also implied that their reputation depended on their hospital's success.

China has mostly limited the development of institutions to the Communist Party, the state and the market. It has expanded the areas subject to a rules-based legal system very slowly and has resisted the establishment of independent stakeholder organizations. As the regulatory challenges become more complex, the limitations of a reliance on bureaucratic approaches have become clear. Regulatory partnerships are emerging between government and stakeholder groups. Government health facilities play an important role in supervising village doctors. The FDRAs in the two counties have established pharmaceutical associations to mobilize the network of drug sellers. This kind of partnership strengthens the regulatory agency's capacity to enforce rules. It also increases the capacity of stakeholders to influence the state in favour of their narrow interests.

One important issue in the health sector is the role of doctors and other skilled personnel. Mature health systems have well-established institutional arrangements to regulate health worker behaviour and mediate decisions about income and status. China does not have such arrangements. One possible reason for the resistance by the health sector to the loss of its right to earn surpluses from the sale of drugs and use of medical equipment is the lack of a trusted system for determining health worker income. However, the reliance on sale of drugs and of diagnostic tests has eroded trust between health workers and clients. The Chinese health sector may eventually need institutional arrangements for encouraging high-quality care and for establishing appropriate levels of health worker pay.

No institutions specifically express the viewpoints of service users. The government has attempted to address this problem by testing popular perceptions through complaint lines and opinion polls. In practice, very few complaints have been received. However, other evidence suggests that people have only limited trust in health system providers. They may also have limited trust in the capacity of the above-mentioned agencies to change the situation.

The institutional arrangements documented in this chapter have emerged as piecemeal responses to emergent problems. Some agencies have parallel responsibilities. No single agency has an overview of the development of the health sector. The study city is preparing its first regional health resource plan, but this will probably focus largely on infrastructure. The supervisory body of the NCMS schemes brings together representatives of a number of key government agencies, but the focus is largely on hospital care. Understandings of health system development by local decision-makers are fragmented and piecemeal. There is a lack of a systematic analysis of the interests of the different stakeholders and the ways they organize to promote them. There is also no forum at which stakeholders can negotiate arrangements that meet their competing interests.

The government's 2009 announcement of major new health system initiatives and large increases in public funding of rural health services marked a new stage in the development of China's health sector. The performance of a county's health services has been made an important criterion for the assessment of the overall performance of local government leaders. At the time of the study, the counties had demonstrated a lot of progress with institution building since the central government had first acknowledged the existence of serious problems in the rural health system. However, the incompleteness of the institutional arrangements and the lack of a systematic analysis of the dynamics of institutional development still had an important influence on the health system's performance. County governments need to do a lot more to create a trustworthy and trusted health system. Their capacity to build these institutions will strongly influence the outcome of the present health reform efforts.

Acknowledgements

The authors acknowledge the strong support by the Chinese Health Economics Institute, the Guangxi Provincial Health Department and the governments of the two study counties, without which the study would have been impossible. They would also like to thank Pei Xiaomei, Bruno Meessen, Henry Lucas and other researchers in the Hospitals in Change Project, who made important contributions to every aspect of the study. The research was funded by a grant by the European Union to the Hospitals in Change Project. Additional resources were provided for the final writing up by the DFID-supported Future Health Systems Research Programme Consortium. The contents of the chapter are the sole responsibility of the authors.

References

Bloom, G. (2005) 'Health policy during China's transition to a market economy', in R. Gauld (ed.) *Comparative Health Policy in the Asia-Pacific*, Open University Press, Maidenhead, UK

Bloom, G. (2011) 'Building institutions for an effective health system: lessons from China's experience with rural health reform', *Social Science and Medicine*, 72 (8): 1302–1309

Bloom, G., Standing, H. and Lloyd, R. (2008) 'Markets, information asymmetry and health care: towards new social contracts', *Social Science and Medicine*, 66 (10): 2076–2087

Central Committee of the Communist Party of China and the State Council (CCCPC) (2009) *Opinions of the Central Committee of the Communist Party of China and the State Council on Deepening the Health Care System Reform*, CCCPC, Beijing

Eggleston, K., Li, L., Meng, Q., Lindelow, M. and Wagstaff, A. (2008) 'Health service delivery in China: a literature review', *Health Economics*, 17: 149–165

Fang, J. (2008) 'The Chinese health care regulatory institutions in an era of transition', *Social Science and Medicine*, 66 (4): 952–962

Gilson, L. (2003) 'Trust and the development of health care as a social institution', *Social Science and Medicine*, 56 (7): 1453–1468

Gong, Y., Wilkes, A. and Bloom, G. (1997) 'Health human resource development in rural China', *Health Policy and Planning*, 12 (4): 320–328

Huang, Y. (1995) 'Administrative monitoring in China', *China Quarterly*, 143: 837–838

Li, P. (2002) 'Changes in social stratification in China since the reform', *Social Sciences in China*, 23 (1): 42–47

Lieberthal, K. and Oksenberg, M. (1988) *Policy Making in China: Leaders, Structures, and Processes*, Princeton University Press, Princeton, NJ

Liu, C. (2003) 'The battle against SARS: a Chinese story', *Australian Health Review*, 26 (3): 3–13

Lubman, S. (1999) *Bird in a Cage: Legal Reform in China after Mao*, Stanford University Press, Stanford, CA

Mackintosh, M. (1999) 'Informal regulation: a conceptual framework and application to decentralized health care systems', in M. Mackintosh and R. Roy (eds), *Economic Decentralization and Public Management Reform*, Edward Elgar, Cheltenham, UK

North, D. C. (2005) *Understanding the Process of Economic Change*, Princeton University Press, Princeton, NJ

Oi, J. (1999) *Rural China Takes Off: Institutional Foundations of Economic Reform*, University of California Press, Berkeley

Pei, X. and Bloom, G. (2011) 'Balancing efficiency and legitimacy: institutional changes and rural health organization in China', *Social Policy and Administration*, 45 (6): 662–677

Tang, S. and Bloom, G. (2000) 'Decentralizing rural health services: a case study in China', *International Journal of Health Planning and Management*, 15 (3): 189–200

Tomba, L. (2001) *Paradoxes of Labour Reform: Chinese Labour Theory and Practice from Socialism to Market*, RoutledgeCurzon, London

Tsai, K. (2002) *Back-Alley Banking: Private Entrepreneurs in China*, Cornell University Press, Ithaca, NY

Wagstaff, A., Yip, W., Lindelow, M. and Hsiao, W. (2009a) 'China's health system and its reform: a review of recent studies', *Health Economics*, 18: S7–S23

Wagstaff, A., Lindelow, M., Wang, S. and Zhang, S. (2009b) *Reforming China's Rural Health System*, World Bank, Washington, DC

Wang, Y. (2008) 'The policy process and context of the new cooperative medical scheme and financial assistance in China', in B. Meessen, X. Pei, B. Criel and G. Bloom (eds) *Health and Social Protection: Experiences from China, Cambodia and Lao PDR*, Institute of Tropical Medicine, Antwerp

Wu, H., Ren, J., Fang, L. and Cui, X. (2005) 'General report of case studies on THCs in rural China', unpublished report for INCO-funded Hospitals in Change Project

Zhang, Z., Fang, L. and Bloom, G. (2009) 'The rural health protection system in China', in V. Lin, Y. Guo, D. Legge and Q. Wu (eds) *Health Policy in Transition: The Challenges for China*, Peking University Medical Press, Beijing

Zweig, D. (2000) 'The externalities of development: can new political institutions manage rural conflict?', in E. Perry and M. Selden (eds) *Chinese Society: Change, Conflict and Resistance*, Routledge, London

6 Informal markets in sexual and reproductive health services and commodities in rural and urban Bangladesh

Hilary Standing, Sabina Faiz Rashid and Owasim Akram

Introduction

Little attention has been paid to informal medical markets for sexual and reproductive health (SRH) services in developing countries, yet recent empirical research in both rural and urban Bangladesh shows that they are substantial and has revealed significant resort by poor men and women to informal providers of SRH services. This chapter examines the characteristics of the informal market for these services, showing how supply and demand mutually reinforce the development of this flourishing market, especially in the absence of high-quality formal provision. Building on a mapping of all health service providers in three areas in Bangladesh, it describes the types of providers, their demographic characteristics and the kinds of treatment they provide, noting any rural and urban diversity. It examines the nature of demand for services and the perspectives of users on these informal providers. Gender particularly influences patterns of resort and the development of specialist niches among providers. Men in both rural and urban areas spend considerable amounts of money in the informal market for consultations, particularly consultations focusing on psychosexual anxieties. For women, these providers are often the only resort for treatment of neglected and sometimes stigmatized SRH conditions.

The chapter also notes how these local markets are increasingly infused with global influences on sexual and reproductive health-seeking behaviour, particularly the influx of unregulated pharmaceutical products into informal pharmacies. The globalization of local markets creates additional complexities in relation to policy messages with regard to appropriate responses to informal markets for SRH services.

Background

The Bangladesh health sector

Bangladesh's public health service delivery system is hierarchically structured from the national level to the village level. In rural areas there are three tiers of health institutions comprising district hospitals, sub-district (upazila) health complexes and community (union) level health and family welfare centres which provide different public healthcare services. SRH services provided at sub-district and community level consist of maternal and child health services and family planning. The health workforce similarly comprises different-level providers, with medical doctors mainly based at district and sub-district facilities, and a range of paramedical staff – family welfare visitors (FWVs), health inspectors (HIs), medical assistants, sub-assistant community medical officers (SACMOs), pharmacists, medical technologists and birth attendants – at community level (Mridha *et al.*, 2009).

Private health care is an important component of the national healthcare system of Bangladesh, providing services to those sections of the population who can afford the services and are ready to pay for them. Since the 1950s, private practice by public-sector physicians has been important in Bangladesh because of the small number of private-sector physicians. No clear policy covers this practice (Khan, 1995, p. 1). The Fifth Five Year Plan reported that 'a large number of government employed doctors carry on private practice in the health sector' (Government of Bangladesh, 1998, p. 481). A study reported that 33 per cent of doctors with a Bachelor of Medicine, Bachelor of Surgery (MBBS) degree and 51 per cent of specialists who are public-sector personnel are involved in private practice (ORG-Marg Quest, 2000, p. 10). This pattern reflects both the shortage of qualified health personnel in the country and the opportunities private practice provides to increase earnings.

Other providers cross the public–private boundary, offering services (including diagnostics) from private clinics while being in government service. Private health care also cuts across the formal and informal sectors, ranging from traditional treatments to modern allopathic medicine. Informal healthcare workers are those healthcare providers operating outside the formal rules regulating the practice and conduct of health workers. Practitioners include village doctors, with or without formal training, and highly qualified practitioners working in relatively formal settings in private clinics (Rahman, 2007). As noted, the public sector provides limited services or support for SRH, and a large and mainly informal market has developed to fill the gap.

A recent survey in Bangladesh found that there were only 0.58 qualified health workers for every 1,000 population, which is far short of the optimal 2.5 workers per 1,000 recommended by the World Health Organization (WHO). Of these, only 16 per cent are located in rural areas. It is estimated that more than 85 per cent of the population is treated by informal providers who fill the huge gap in health human resources (Bangladesh Health Watch Report, 2008). They include homoeopaths, birth attendants, village doctors ('quacks'), unregistered pharmacists and faith healers (Omaswa, 2006; World Bank, 2003). Traditional healers and village doctors often advise on family planning methods, pregnancy, STDs, diarrhoea and acute respiratory infections. It is estimated that a majority of those suffering from sexually transmitted infections (STIs) are treated by medicine sellers (Ahmed and Hossain, 2009).

The study context: research design and methodology

The study was conducted in three sites: Chittagong, the second-largest city of Bangladesh (Matijharna slum – urban, south-east), Rangpur (Gangachara Upazila – rural, north-west) and Sylhet (Jagannathpur Upazila – rural, north-east; upazilas are sub-districts). The last recorded census figures give a population of 192,336 for Gangachara and 188,139 for Jagannathpur (BBS, 2006). Matijharna slum (the fourteenth ward of Chittagong City Corporation) has an estimated population of 69,865 (BBS, 2006). Structured and semi-structured questionnaires were administered to 311 ever married men (meaning men who had been married, whether or not they were currently married) and 312 ever married women in the age range 15–49 years and 303 providers, covering at least 100 from each of the three sites.

Data were collected in three phases from July 2008 to January 2009. Respondents were selected from every fifth household (in the rural setting) or tenth household (in the urban site, owing to high household density) starting from a central point and continuing until the desired sample size was reached. Selection was done to avoid any possibility of selecting two respondents from the same or nearest household, or surveying people who would be very well known to each other, given the sensitivity of the topic. Interviews were conducted in a place convenient for the interviewee without the presence of friends, neighbours or family members. The male and female questionnaires generated information on socio-demographic status; community SRH concerns, their causes and perceived severity; self-experience of SRH concerns suffered within the past twelve months, along with health-seeking history; knowledge about sexual and reproductive health problems, family planning issues, abortion and contraceptive use; and information about the providers they used.

For the provider part of the study, the providers were first mapped to capture all providers of SRH services in the three sites. All markets (*haat*), fixed shops and major social gathering points of eight unions of Gangachhara Upazila in Rangpur and nine unions of Jagannathpur Upazila in Sunamganj were mapped. For the urban site (Chittagong), mapping was conducted only in the fourteenth ward (the smallest urban administrative unit), corresponding to Matijharna slum, where the survey of SRH service users took place. The list of providers was generated from detailed geographical mapping and from information about providers reported in the surveys from the three sites. For the mapping, a short questionnaire was designed covering age, type of service, education, main occupation, SRH services offered and referral practice if any. On the basis of this questionnaire, the list was then matched with the providers list generated from the surveys of female and male users. In each study site the research team compared lists and excluded possible duplicate names by matching the names and addresses, along with the type of services, with information received from users. It is, however, possible that some duplicate cases exist, as a few were identified by designations such as 'Rahim's wife', rather than by their own names.

The mapping of all sexual and reproductive health service providers from the three sites who were found to be treating SRH conditions revealed 925 active providers, of whom 560 (60.5 per cent) were male and 311 (33.6 per cent) were female. The remaining ones (5.8 per cent) were identified as various clinics, hospitals or organizations providing services for SRH. From this mapping, 303 were selected for a survey covering at least 100 providers from each study site, of whom 62 per cent were male and 38 per cent female. The sample of providers covered at least one of every type of provider and location of service provision, including qualified doctors, homoeopaths, government hospitals, non-governmental organizations (NGOs), clinics, private clinics, village doctors (sometimes called rural medical practitioners or *palli chikitsok*), faith healers, *kabiraj, hakim* (herbalists), family planning workers, medical assistants, health assistants, pharmacists, unlicensed drug sellers, birth attendants (traditional and skilled) and street-based medicine sellers. The providers' survey questionnaire generated information on socio-demographic profile, service pattern and experience related to SRH services, knowledge and perception about male and female SRH concerns, and information on fees charged, referral practices and follow-up, family planning issues, menstrual regulation (MR) and abortion practices.

The marketplace for SRH services

In this section we look at how the market for SRH services operates, focusing on the types of providers and the nature of the demand for their services. As noted, it is not easy to draw a clear distinction between formal and informal providers, as the boundaries between public and private, formal and informal, in the Bangladesh health system are blurred and the system is heavily marketized. Across the range of providers, many working in the public sector also operate as market-based independent providers. Doctors employed in government facilities generally have their own private practices in the afternoon and evening. Other health workers employed in public facilities also provide 'private' services. Informal payment demands and referrals across this boundary by public-sector providers are common.

In Bangladesh there are several regulatory and statutory bodies that have a mandate to oversee training and development of qualified health professionals, ensure the provision of standardized health services to the population, protect their right to health and ensure access to quality health services. The main statutory bodies are the Bangladesh Medical and Dental Council (BMDC), the Bangladesh Nursing Council (BNC), the State Medical Faculty (SMF), the Bangladesh Pharmacy Council (BPC) and the Bangladesh Board of Unani and Ayurvedic Systems of Medicine (BBUASM). Registration and oversight of private medical facilities are the responsibility of the Director General of Health Services. The Parliamentary Standing Committee on health plays an oversight role on behalf of the government and citizens. According to a recent study on health-sector governance in Bangladesh, the various regulatory and oversight bodies function poorly, owing to politicization and lack of accountability (Bangladesh Health Watch Report, 2009). Rules are not enforced and disciplinary and redress mechanisms are either absent or non-functioning.

The legal and regulatory environment is also ambiguous in relation to oversight of informal providers. For example, the SMF was established during British rule for the purpose of developing and overseeing new cadres of front-line health staff, and for a short period, between 1979 and 1983, provided authorized training and certification to village doctors (*palli chikitshok*). These are the forerunners of the current village doctors, or 'quacks', who are no longer an officially sanctioned cadre but are an established feature of the informal healthcare market in Bangladesh. Similarly, practitioners of Unani and Ayurvedic medicine are in theory certified and regulated by the BBUASM but in practice there is little oversight at local level. Many other practitioners do not fall under any of the current statutory bodies. The informal market is a fluid and dynamic concept in relation both to the status of many providers and to the often routinely marketized transactions between formal as well as informal providers and users.

Characteristics of the providers

The 925 formal and informal providers of SRH-related services found in the mapping survey providers were relatively evenly split between the three sites (Rangpur 30.6 per cent, Sunamganj 33.6 per cent, Chittagong 35.8 per cent). As the population of the urban site was less than half of that of the other two sites, this indicates the much higher density of providers in the urban area. Table 6.1 shows the distribution by site and gender. Out of these, fifty-four were facilities which spanned public, commercial and NGO clinics and hospitals, Ayurvedic clinics and shrines, and which were noted by users as popular sources of SRH services. Overall, of the individual providers, one-third were women but the proportion was higher in the urban study site. Notably, a much higher number of formal facilities providing services were found in the urban study site.

Table 6.2 gives a detailed breakdown of types of provider or facility by study site in descending order of numbers. Again, rural–urban differences are apparent. Almost half the qualified doctors and the majority of the formal medical facilities are in the urban site while the majority of the village doctors ('quacks') are in the two rural sites. The 'formal' health sector in the Rangpur site is mainly represented by a few front-line health and family planning workers, including some NGO-based staff.

Table 6.1 Distribution of total sexual and reproductive health (SRH) providers by site and gender

Type	Total		Rangpur		Sunamgang		Chittagong	
	No.	*%*	*No.*	*%*	*No.*	*%*	*No.*	*%*
Male	560	60.5	205	72.4	192	61.7	163	49.2
Female	311	33.6	77	27.2	108	34.7	126	38.1
Facilities – public, private, NGO, other systems	54	5.8	1	0.4	11	3.5	42	12.7
Total	**925**		**283**		**311**		**331**	

Table 6.2 Types of provider by study site

Type of providers	Total		Rangpur		Sunamganj		Chittagong	
	No.	%	No.	%	No.	%	No.	%
Qualified physicians	233	25.2	31	11.0	83	26.7	119	36.0
Traditional medicine practitioners	229	24.8	96	33.9	71	22.8	62	18.7
Birth attendants (traditional and skilled)	183	19.8	44	15.5	73	23.5	66	19.9
Homoeopaths	83	9.0	37	13.1	30	9.6	16	4.8
Village doctors (*palli chikitshok*)	68	7.4	35	12.4	29	9.3	4	1.2
Drugstore salespeople	60	6.5	24	8.5	14	4.5	22	6.6
Biomedical paraprofessionals	41	4.4	14	4.9	11	3.5	16	4.8
Community health workers	25	2.7	0	0.0	0	0.0	25	7.6
Trained nurses	3	0.3	2	0.7	0	0.0	1	0.3
Total	**925**		**283**		**311**		**331**	

Of the total number of individual providers mapped, more than two-thirds (633) said that they provided SRH-related services to both women and men; 96 provided SRH-related services only to men and 196 reported that they provided SRH services only to women.

Table 6.3 shows the types and numbers of the 303 individual providers that were surveyed in detail and whether they are employed in a public facility. Of these providers, 63 (20.8 per cent) were government service providers. None of the birth attendants in the survey were associated with public facilities, although they have received some formal training. All the providers employed in a public facility reported that they were also practising privately. This indicates the widespread nature of unsanctioned, informalized practice by government employees.

Table 6.4 gives information on the primary place of practice of the surveyed group of providers. Less than a third of them were primarily hospital or clinic based, with a high proportion based in pharmacies or drugstores.

The 303 providers had an average age of 46 years and an average of 17.6 years' experience as a provider. Twenty-five per cent reported having institutionally recognized degrees and medical training, and 63 per cent were informal providers who had not received any formally recognized training but claimed they learned by working with their employers or receiving guidance from others, while the remaining 12 per cent had had no training, formal or informal. In terms of education, 15 per cent of the total 303 providers claimed to hold a Bachelor of Medicine, Bachelor of Surgery (MBBS) degree, while the rest of the providers (13 per cent) reported studying up to college level (Bachelor or Master's level), with 34 per cent reportedly completing ten to twelve years of education. Twenty-two

Table 6.3 Categorization of providers

SL	Type	Total providers (n = 303)		Involved with government facilities (n = 303)	
		No.	Percentage	No.	Percentage
1.	Traditional medicine practitioners	70	23.1	–	–
2.	Birth attendants (traditional and skilled)	51	16.8	–	–
3.	Physicians[a]	44	14.5	31	10.2
4.	Drugstore salespeople	33	10.9	–	–
5.	Allopathic paraprofessionals	30	9.9	30	10.0
6.	Village doctors	30	9.9	–	–
7.	Homoeopaths	30	9.9	–	–
8.	Community health workers	11	3.6	–	–
9.	Nurses	4	1.3	2	0.6
Total		**303**	**100.0**	**63**	**20.8**

Notes: 1 = faith healers (*hujur*), street healers (*kabiraj, Ojha, Boiddo, Totka*), herbal, Ayurvedic;
5 = family welfare assistant (FWA), family welfare visitor (FWV), health assistant (HA),
sub-assistant community medical officer (SACMO), medical assistant (MA); 8 = NGO paramedics/
health workers, community mobilizers, outreach workers; 9 = nurses (two working in government
clinics and two in NGO clinics). The categorization of providers is taken from the categories in
Bangladesh Health Watch Report (2008).

a   Refers to MBBS-level medical doctors.

Table 6.4 Primary place of practice

Practising place	No.	%
Pharmacy	65	21.4
Government hospital/clinic	63	20.8
Own chamber	52	17.2
Own residence	49	16.2
On-call service	32	10.6
NGO hospital/clinic	15	5.0
Private clinic	9	3.0
Mobile (market/street)	9	3.0
Mosque	5	1.7
Shrine	4	1.3
Total	**303**	

per cent had studied below Class 10, and 16 per cent of the surveyed providers did
not have any formal education at all. Aside from formal medical training, providers
reported learning their knowledge and skills from a range of sources, including
inspirational or dream-based learning, inheritance from family members, religious
books, and learning by experience (working closely with relatives or colleagues).
Most said they obtained their skills informally through experience: 'learning by

doing, watching others'. Traditional healers generally got their knowledge through divine revelations (dreams) and learning from their fathers and senior elders.

Of the 303 providers, 75 per cent said that healing was their main profession, while 25 per cent practised it as a side business. This latter group largely comprised informal providers who had other employment or who farmed or ran other businesses. It was not possible to collect systematic information on providers' incomes from treating SRH concerns, but 35 per cent reported that they did not charge any money for their services. The majority of these were either government providers or NGO workers, and this does not take into account the informal payments that are commonly demanded in government facilities. Thirty-three per cent said that they charged a fee for their services, while 15 per cent said they received gifts in kind for services rendered, and 13 per cent said they did not charge for consultations but charged for the costs of medicines. Four per cent said that they already received a salary elsewhere and so did not charge a fee, and 1 per cent did not respond to the question. It was estimated that on average providers see sixteen male patients and fourteen female patients per day, of which two male patients and five female patients present with SRH problems.

There was evidence of links between different types of providers through referrals, with the majority (77 per cent) claiming that they referred patients with SRH-related concerns to other specialized providers in the case of conditions that they could not treat. Out of the 208 providers, 151 said that they do not provide treatment for one or more SRH conditions and refer patients with these conditions to other formal and informal providers.

The majority of responses (85 per cent) cited the superior experience of the provider as the main reason for referral, while 25 per cent of the responses mentioned knowing the provider personally and another 23 per cent cited their local popularity as a provider. A few (3 per cent) mentioned that the provider they referred to gave better service to the poor.

Table 6.5 Referral patterns of providers for SRH conditions

Type (n = 151, multiple response)	*Fre. (%)*
Allopathic doctors (not specified whether formal or informal)	50
MBBS doctors sitting in private chambers	31.1
Government hospitals	9.3
Kabiraj	8
Homoeopath	4

Men's and women's use of the SRH marketplace

Characteristics of the service users

Of the 312 ever married women interviewed from the three sites, the average age was 31 years, while the average age for the men was 36 years. Table 6.6 shows the

Table 6.6 Age distribution of male and female respondents

Age	Men		Women	
	No.	*%*	*No.*	*%*
<20	3	1.0	22	7.1
21–30	106	34.1	141	45.2
31–40	114	36.7	113	36.2
41+	88	28.3	36	11.5
Total	**311**		**312**	

age breakdown by gender. The women clustered more in the younger age groups, with nearly half of the female respondents falling into the 21–30 age group and twenty-two of them below the age of 20. The average length of married life for women was fourteen years, and 70 per cent had married before reaching 18 years of age; 28.5 per cent had married by the time they were 15 years old. The average length of married life of the men was twelve years, reflecting their later age at marriage.

In terms of educational status, 39 per cent of the women did not have any formal schooling, 31 per cent had some experience of primary-level schooling (years 1 to 5) and 28 per cent had high-school-level schooling (years 6 to 9). Only 2 per cent of the women had completed Secondary School Certificate (SSC – year 10) or studied more. Of the men, 34 per cent of respondents did not have any formal education; 32 per cent had had experience of primary-level schooling. Thirty-one per cent had experience of high-school-level schooling up to level 10 and only 3 per cent had experience of secondary school or more.

The average monthly household income of the women respondents was Bangladesh taka (BDT) 6,668 (equivalent to US$96) and that of the men was BDT 7,105 (equivalent to US$105). Twenty-five per cent of the women and 26.7 per cent of the men and their households were in the lowest income quintile, earning below BDT 3,000 or US$43 per month. Of these, almost half (see Table 6.7) belonged to the rural area of Rangpur, which is one of the areas of the country affected by seasonal food insecurity (*monga*).

Across the three research sites, 87 per cent of the women did not work outside the home, 3 per cent reported holding private or government jobs, and the remaining 10 per cent were involved in small-scale activities such as tailoring and other micro-enterprises (selling food and livestock), rearing animals, and day labouring and domestic service. Of the men, 24 per cent reported involvement with small or medium-sized businesses; 20 per cent of respondents reported that they were working as day labourers; 14 per cent were involved with farming; 13 per cent were rickshaw pullers; 11.5 per cent were masons, carpenters, mechanics, cooks, waiters or self-employed; 7 per cent held formal private or government positions; 6 per cent drove buses or auto-rickshaws; 2.3 per cent were involved in fishing; and 1.5 per cent reported as unemployed.

Table 6.7 Income in quintiles (%)

Income quintiles[a]	Region							
	All sites		Rangpur		Sunamganj		Chittagong	
	Male (n = 311)	Female (n = 312)	Male (n = 107)	Female (n = 101)	Male (n = 104)	Female (n = 109)	Male (n = 100)	Female (n = 102)
Lowest	26.7	25.0	44.9	43.6	22.1	11.0	12.0	21.6
Second	15.4	12.8	20.6	15.8	16.3	11.0	9.0	11.8
Middle	19.0	14.4	16.8	12.9	18.3	14.7	22.0	15.7
Fourth	23.2	19.6	10.3	17.8	20.2	15.6	40.0	25.5
Highest	15.8	18.2	7.5	9.9	23.1	47.7	17.0	25.5

Note
a   Lowest = <3,000 taka; second = 3,001–4,000 taka; middle = 4,001–5,000 taka; fourth = 5,001–8,000 taka; highest = >8,000 taka.

SRH concerns taken to providers

Both men and women reported high levels of problems, and resorted to different providers for SRH concerns. There were marked gender differences in the responses. Of the male respondents, 151 (48.6 per cent) said that they had suffered or were still suffering from at least one SRH concern over the previous twelve months, of whom 90 (59.6 per cent) had sought and received treatment. Among the women, 273 (87.5 per cent) reported at least one SRH concern and of these, 152 (55.7 per cent) had sought and received treatment.

The high level of concern about sexual performance and sex-related conditions and anxieties reported by men (Table 6.8) is notable.

Women's self-reported concerns (Table 6.9) included a significant number associated with menstruation and aspects of maternal health, which are largely neglected by the formal healthcare system. They also include a number of conditions that are subject to shame or stigma and that were mentioned by many providers as conditions for which women commonly seek treatment, such as smelly discharge, genital sores and warts, and pain or discomfort during sexual intercourse.

For both men and women, the primary self-reported SRH health concerns are ones that are neglected in government health service provision. The SRH component of the essential health services package in Bangladesh is focused on basic antenatal and delivery services for women, along with family planning. Little curative care is provided and there is no provision for men's SRH. Family planning does not target men. Further, both women and men reported frequent concerns with more culturally defined conditions, particularly white discharge for women and semen loss and other sexual anxieties for men. These concerns are found commonly across South Asia (Kakar, 1996; Collumbien *et al.*, 1998). The self-report data reveal a high level of demand for SRH services and information, a

Table 6.8 SRH concerns reported by men

Types of concerns (n =151; multiple responses)	Fre. (%)
Shortened duration of sexual intercourse/premature ejaculation	33.8
Frequent urination or incontinence	26.5
Loss of semen before and after urination	23.8
Burning or pain when urinating	23.2
Nocturnal emissions	15.2
Unable to maintain an erection/impotence	14.6
Itching or burning	12.6
Ekshira/hernia/hydrocele	9.3
Ejaculation before coitus	7.9
Anxieties about the penis or other parts of the body	5.3
Discharge of pus from the penis	2.6
Pain during sexual intercourse	2.6
Piles	2.0
Loss of semen	1.3
Worries about masturbation	1.3
Open sores	1.3
Pain in the testicles	0.7
Bumps or sores anywhere on the penis	0.7

Table 6.9 SRH concerns reported by women

Types of concerns (n = 273; multiple responses)	Fre. (%)
White discharge	57.9
Lower back pain	43.6
Lower abdominal pain	34.4
Painful or burning sensations when urinating	24.5
Irregular menstruation	24.5
No bleeding during menstruation or reduced bleeding	20.1
Irritation and itching of the female genital area	15.8
Prolapse (uterus coming out through the vagina)	13.6
Unable to hold in urine/little drops of urine come out when sneezing or coughing	12.8
Discomfort or pain during intercourse	10.9
Excessive bleeding during menstruation	8.4
Low sexual desire	8.4
Bleeding between menstrual periods	5.9
Miscarriage	5.1
Open sores anywhere on the genitals	4.0
Infertility (unable to conceive)	2.9
Smelly vaginal discharge	2.9
Genital warts (single or multiple)	2.6
Bleeding during vaginal intercourse	1.8
Abortion	1.8
Unable to have complete sexual satisfaction	1.8
Unable to become aroused or maintain arousal during sexual activity	1.1

demand that is being met substantially by the market. Tables 6.10 and 6.11 show the most-used service providers for SRH services as identified by men and women respectively.

Village doctors are notably popular with both men and women. Men also commonly use pharmacies and street-based drug sellers. Government services and qualified doctors are used more by women, probably as a consequence of the bias in government services towards maternal and child health and family planning, and also the greater resort among urban women in particular to private obstetricians and gynaecologists. Resort to MBBS doctors refers generally to privately practising doctors understood by respondents to be qualified (i.e. to be known as MBBS). However, these doctors' qualifications could not always be verified and it is likely that at least some of them were village doctors. Information on patterns

Table 6.10 Most-used SRH service provider: men

Type of provider	Fre.	%
Village doctor	68	21.9
Drug-seller/pharmacy	57	18.3
MBBS doctor	47	15.1
Homoeopath	31	10.0
Kabiraj/hakim	22	7.1
Government health centre	11	3.5
Roadside healer	3	1.0
Faith healer	2	0.6
Private hospital	1	0.3
Don't know	69	22.2
Total	**311**	

Table 6.11 Most-used SRH service provider: women

Type of provider	Fre.	%
MBBS doctor	79	25.3
Village doctor	75	24.0
Government health centre/hospital	36	11.5
Drug-seller/pharmacist	24	7.7
Faith healer (*hujur*)	21	6.7
Homoeopath	18	5.8
Family planning worker	14	4.5
Traditional birth attendant	10	3.2
Private hospital	7	2.2
Kabiraj/herbalist	6	1.9
NGO health worker	6	1.9
NGO clinic	4	1.3
Friends/relatives	1	0.3
Don't know	11	3.5
Total	**312**	

of treatment seeking reveals pluralistic behaviour switching between different types of provider until a satisfactory outcome is obtained, and with no consistent pattern of resort across the formal–informal spectrum. Choice of provider is determined by several factors, but the two most commonly cited are the provider's reputation locally, which particularly covers their ready availability and respectful behaviour to patients, and their willingness to keep their charges low. These are encapsulated in one respondent's comments about a well-regarded village doctor: 'Dr Shoyeb [village doctor] comes to the home even if he is called at dead of night on emergency. He doesn't charge a poor man and takes only the price of medicine.'

External influences on local markets

The research revealed a thriving informal market, particularly in services and commodities for addressing sexual concerns. Some of this is traditional in the sense that there has always been an important niche for local providers in treating culturally grounded conditions such as semen loss in men (Collumbien *et al.*, 1998; Collumbien and Hawkes, 2000). Providers were asked about the treatments they used for sexual performance anxieties. Of the 208 providers of SRH services to men, 142 said that they provide treatment or medication for enhancing sexual performance. Of the 265 providers of SRH services to women, 97 said that they provide treatment or medication to women for enhancing sexual performance. These practitioners were fairly evenly spread across the categories of provider. Table 6.12 shows the kinds of treatments they provide.

This indicates the mix of traditional and more recent responses, with providers offering widely available pharmaceuticals and vitamins as treatments. The study found evidence of more global influences on this market for sexual health aids. Rapid urbanization, an increasingly mobile labour force of low-income men and women, and the accompanying transformation of gender relations in both rural and urban areas have produced a burgeoning sex industry, an influx of pornography and sex clinics, and private or informal providers selling 'sexual medicines'

Table 6.12 Treatments for sexual performance anxieties (multiple responses)

Treatments reported by providers	For men (%) (n = 142 providers)	For women (%) (n = 97 providers)
Vitamins	40	57.7
Pharmaceutical drugs	38	23.7
Herbal tonics	32.4	16.5
Homoeopathic medicines	17	7.2
Medicinal plants	15	10.3
Oil/cream massaging	13	3.1
Psychological counselling	8	6.2
Amulets	7	6.2
Other	24	10.3

which men at all income levels increasingly have access to. The popular media and both local and international pornography that are accessed through satellite television, DVD players, the internet, mobile phones, magazines and news items, not available on this scale even a decade ago, have provided new images with which to imagine and perform relationships, sexual behaviour, intimacy and sexualities. Local and international pornography and an informal market economy of health providers are facilitating different notions of male and female desire in a context where there is still little public acknowledgement and open discussion of sexual health. This will have implications for the sexual and reproductive health of men and women.

Conclusion

In this chapter we have described the flourishing market, much of it informal, for SRH services. Poor people in both rural and urban areas were found to consult a wide range of providers for SRH concerns and to pay for these services. This market flourishes for several reasons. First, health services are poorly regulated and overseen in Bangladesh, leading to many government providers working privately and encouraging patients to use private services. Second, there are absolute and relative shortages of qualified providers in Bangladesh, particularly in rural and poor urban areas. Third, government services provide little in the way of SRH services aside from family planning and basic delivery care, leaving the informal and formal market to fill the vacuum. Fourth, and related to this, the study revealed major gender-related demands for services and information that formal service provision does not fulfil. Men reported many SRH concerns and anxieties, including possible sexually transmitted infections, that are poorly or inadequately addressed in government services, while women used market-based providers for neglected or stigmatized SRH conditions, including childbirth-related morbidity. The study also noted the relative importance of culturally specific syndromes in SRH, which have generally been the province of informal providers. At the same time, there is evidence that suggests the market is responding to external and global influences, including widespread availability of over-the-counter pharmaceuticals and the rise of new sources of information on SRH from the internet and satellite television.

This complex and changing market in SRH services raises considerable policy challenges. There are aspects that would benefit from stronger regulation and oversight, such as inappropriate drug therapy, and from improved training of professional and paramedic cadres. But greatly improved formal-sector provision of a broader range of professionalized SRH services in the context of Bangladesh's considerable shortages of health workers will not be achieved soon. Further, the very broad and gendered nature of the demand for SRH services suggests that other pathways to meeting some of these needs may be more appropriate. These could be in the form of high-quality assured provision of information, particularly on sexual health, through a range of channels, and support for improving the knowledge and skills of trusted popular providers.

References

Ahmed, S. M. and Hossain, M. A. (2009) 'Informal sector providers in Bangladesh: how equipped they are to provide rational health care?', *Health Policy and Planning*, 24 (6): 467–478

Bangladesh Bureau of Statistics (BBS) (2006) *Population Census – 2001*, Zilla Series (Rangpur, Sunamganj and Chittagong), Planning Division, Government of Bangladesh, Dhaka

Bangladesh Health Watch Report (2008) *The State of Health in Bangladesh in 2007; Health Workforce in Bangladesh: Who Constitutes the Healthcare System?*, Bangladesh Health Watch, BRAC University School of Public Health, Dhaka

Bangladesh Health Watch Report (2009) *How Healthy Is Health Sector Governance?*, University Press, Dhaka

Collumbien, M. and Hawkes, S. (2000) 'Missing men's messages: does the reproductive health approach respond to men's sexual health needs?', *Culture, Health and Sexuality*, 2 (2): 135–150

Collumbien, M., Bohidar, N., Das, R., Das, B. and Pelto, P. J. (1998) *Male Sexual Health Concerns in Orissa: An Emic Perspective*, AIMS Research Centre, Bhubaneshwar, Orissa

Government of Bangladesh (1998) *The Fifth Five Year Plan 1997–2002*, Planning Commission, Government of Bangladesh, Dhaka

Kakar, S. (1996) *The Indian Psyche*, Viking Penguin India, New Delhi

Khan, M. M. (1995) 'Role of private market in the health sector of Bangladesh: some preliminary discussions', paper presented at a seminar organized by the Centre for Development Research, Dhaka, unpublished

Mridha, M. K., Anwar, I. and Koblinsky, M. (2009) 'Public-sector maternal health programmes and services for rural Bangladesh', *Journal of Health Population and Nutrition*, 27 (2): 124–138

Omaswa, F. (2006) 'Informal health workers – to be encouraged or condemned?', *Bulletin of the World Health Organization*, 84 (2): 83

ORG-Marg Quest (2000) *Report on Medical Practitioners and Pharmacists in Bangladesh*, report prepared for NICARE/the British Council, Dhaka

Rahman, M. (2007) 'The state, the private health care sector and regulation in Bangladesh', *Asia Pacific Journal of Public Administration*, 29 (2): 191–206

World Bank (2003) *Private Sector Assessment for Health, Nutrition and Population (HNP) in Bangladesh*, report no. 27005-BD, World Bank, Washington, DC

7 Improving the performance of patent medicine vendors in Nigeria

Oladimeji Oladepo and Henry Lucas

Introduction

In Nigeria it has long been recognized that those usually described as patent medicine vendors (PMVs) – owners and managers of small shops selling pharmaceuticals and other products – are a major source of health care for dwellers in resource-poor communities, and are often the first source of health care outside the home (Brieger *et al.*, 2007). However, the medical establishment has typically adopted a hostile approach to PMVs, arguing that their lack of training and dependence on the sale of drugs to make a living results in low-quality and possibly dangerous service provision. In particular, it has promoted legislation that tightly restricts the variety of treatments that PMVs can offer. This chapter offers an alternative approach, examining the strength of PMVs and their important role in providing affordable health care in poor rural areas. It takes as a case study the provision of anti-malarial care and demonstrates that, while there are some drawbacks in terms of accuracy and quality of diagnosis and treatment, with the proper infrastructure PMVs can help provide health care in communities where such provision would otherwise be rendered very difficult.

This research is important, given that most discussions about options for global health systems reform have been technocratic in nature, suggesting that organizational arrangements for spreading access to the benefits of medical knowledge are unproblematic and limited only by resource constraints. Not surprisingly, the emphasis has been on 'scaling up' or 'rolling out' effective interventions. A learning approach that combines reflexive and deliberative styles is needed to enable policy-makers and researchers to learn from the past and prepare for the future. Future health systems in developing countries will not meet their goals by simply 'cutting and pasting' interventions developed and tested elsewhere. Instead, influencing how such systems actually work will depend on understanding the increasingly complex and unpredictable interactions of local, national and international actors and trends. This raises particular challenges for those who wish health systems to better serve the most vulnerable populations.

This chapter uses the experiences gained from a case study in Nigeria to contribute to the discourse on evidence-to-policy dynamics and stimulate a reconsideration of options for health systems development. It responds to calls in the literature for further exploration in this area and greater engagement of policy makers in specific areas of health research (Global Forum, 2000). These initiatives have mainly focused on the developed world (COHRED, 1990; Global Forum, 1999; Global Forum, 2000). The Future Health Systems (FHS) consortium project discussed here is in line with the widely expressed need for more innovative methods to understand how the nexus of research and policy impacts on the poor.

Institutional arrangements and health service delivery

The introductory chapter in this book describes how most low- and middle-income countries (LMICs) have pluralistic health systems dominated by market relationships involving diverse types of providers, services and goods (Mackintosh and Koivusalo, 2005; Bloom and Standing, 2001; Berman and Rose, 1996). The extent of marketization often implies that official policies on health have limited relevance to the realities that poor people experience. In many cases the spread of markets has been much faster than the capacity of the state, and other key actors, to establish regulatory arrangements. A large proportion of health market transactions take place outside a legal regulatory framework or in settings where regulatory regimes are poorly implemented, particularly for the poor. There is an increasing divergence in the public sector between the notion of a full-time, salaried public service and the reality of health workers with a variety of livelihood strategies that blur the boundaries between 'public' and 'private' sectors. In addition, present arrangements for certifying health workers as competent and ethical have tended not to focus on the providers most used by the poor. Qualified doctors, and especially medical specialists, primarily serve the better off, while the poor often purchase pharmaceuticals from general stores or unlicensed drug-sellers.

The institutional arrangements of a successful health system embody a series of explicit and implicit 'contracts' that accord service providers and other key actors social status and an appropriate income in exchange for acting in the interests of patients and the broader community (Bloom, 2004; Bloom *et al.*, 2006). These contracts involve both formal rules and informal understandings, and they are underpinned by socially accepted norms of behaviour and internalized rules of conduct. They make possible the complex arrangements necessary for translating expert knowledge into trusted and trustworthy services and managing social arrangements for health finance. In the absence of such contracts, people typically rely on local networks to choose the right provider and protect themselves against exploitation, and on extended families and community-based arrangements to help them cope with the burdens of illness.

The complexity of the Nigerian health system

The 1999 National Health Policy specifies the main functions of each tier of government in primary health care. At the national level the National Council on Health, composed of the federal minister and state commissioners of health, advises on national policies, while the Federal Ministry of Health has responsibility for planning and policy coordination. The state Ministries of Health implement national health programmes and run state health institutions, while the local government authorities deliver health services through primary health care centres and dispensaries controlled by local government councils.

A number of institutional factors contribute to the difficulties experienced in undertaking public health reform and establishing regulatory arrangements that promote the provision of quality services to the poor. First, neither the National Health Policy nor the Constitution of 1999 clearly delineates the roles of the three tiers of government. This has contributed to large variations within and across states in the levels of autonomy granted and responsibilities assigned to local governments in the delivery of primary health care (PHC) services. There are also no consistent established rules relating to the provision of financial assistance from the higher tiers of government or to the manner in which such assistance should be allocated within local government area budgets for PHC services. For example, a World Bank study of PHC delivery argues that continuing problems relating to the non-payment of salaries to PHC workers are often due not to a lack of resources but to the very limited accountability at local government area level in the use of public resources transferred from higher tiers of government (Das Gupta *et al.*, 2004).

Second, Nigeria has a highly pluralistic health system characterized by competing categories of provider whose contributions are not harmonized at the national, state or local government levels. Third, there is a large gap between theory and practice. For example, health staff classified as 'public-sector providers' typically supplement their low salaries from a variety of sources. A range of often conflicting incentives influence their behaviour, with damaging consequences in terms of the ability of the poor to obtain quality services. For example, the greater the average number of months for which staff salaries are not paid in a facility, the greater the probability that essential drugs (chloroquine, paracetamol and antibiotics) will be privately provided by facility staff rather than being facility owned (Das Gupta *et al.*, 2004). The situation is leading to an obvious decline in health services provided, which is probably causing staff to provide services privately in exchange for remuneration from their patients (Khemani, 2004). Public PHC facilities, especially in rural areas, are often in a very poor state of repair, lack basic equipment and essential drugs, and are in many cases staffed by largely unsupervised, minimally trained health workers (Ehiri *et al.*, 2005; Hargreaves, 2002). It is not surprising that utilization rates are low, even when morbidity is high.

Implications for the treatment of malaria

The failures of the PHC system are evident in terms of the treatment of malaria, which is a major cause of illness and death in Nigeria. A recent study found that, contrary to government policy in this area, only 2.3 per cent of anti-malarial drugs dispensed across all outlets in Nigeria are artemisinin-combined therapies (ACTs).

Malaria rates have not declined substantially despite repeated attempts by the public sector to implement malaria treatment and control programmes. With an estimated 57.5 million cases and 225,000 deaths, the country accounted for 25 per cent of the global malaria burden in 2006 (WHO, 2006).The 2008 Demographic and Health Survey findings indicated that 11 per cent of maternal and 30 per cent of under-five deaths were due to malaria (National Population Commission of Nigeria, 2008).

The majority of the population depends on informal markets, primarily PMVs, for malaria treatment. However, these operate in a little understood and poorly regulated market that has been largely unaffected by recent government attempts to improve the quality of primary services, to the extent that increasing levels of sub-standard or fake drugs are a major concern. Understanding this market is particularly important at a time when rising malarial drug resistance has prompted changes in government malaria treatment guidelines, which now recommend the use of more expensive and less available ACTs. The reality for most Nigerians is that the PMV market has been largely unaffected by such policies, and access to quality malaria treatment remains extremely low.

The role of PMVs in the treatment of malaria has received insufficient attention by both government and donors. While the government has indicated its commitment to promote public–private partnership initiatives involving PMVs, it has thus far taken no practical action in pursuit of that commitment. Of particular concern is the non-recognition of PMVs beyond their listing as one category of provider in the national anti-malaria policy. There remains strong resistance among policy-makers and health professionals to working with PMVs, based mainly on a perception that the use of PMVs may result in the provision of inappropriate, ineffective and possibly dangerous drugs, draining the very limited resources of the poor and potentially worsening their condition.

If it were possible radically to improve public provision in the short to medium term, further curtailment of the activities of PMVs might be appropriate. However, this seems a very unlikely outcome. The alternative strategy explored here is to seek a better understanding of the role played by PMVs in the treatment of malaria, and then use that understanding to support and regulate their activities in order to improve the quality of services that they provide.

A conceptual framework

In order to analyse the role of PMVs in diagnosing and treating malaria and other conditions, it is essential to understand both health markets overall and the specific changes taking place within Nigeria. In order to address these, we decided to use the market framework presented in Chapter 1 of this book. At the centre of this framework is the relationship between suppliers and consumers. In our case, this was between health service providers and patients. Those relationships are greatly influenced by a multidimensional and complex environment consisting of formal and informal rules and supporting functions (Figure 7.1). The framework implies that effective strategies to improve the operation of such markets, especially for the

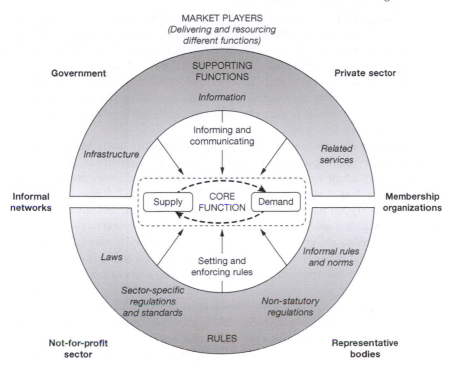

Figure 7.1 Conceptualizing market systems.

Source: Adapted from Elliot *et al.* (2008: figure 3).

poor, need to address the environment for the transactions as well as improving the management of any single organization or intervention. A similar argument is made by Bloom (2001), who emphasizes the importance of assessing the social and political context of health markets, identifying significant power relationships and understanding how these influence market organization and functioning.

The relationship between health providers and patients, which is mainly about transferring the benefits of expert medical knowledge, is characterized by varying degrees of information asymmetry. This problem can be at least partially addressed by effective enforcement of regulations (rules) and the provision of accurate and timely information (supporting function). These may be implemented by a variety of organizations and actors including central or local governments, professional associations and private health companies, and communities, families and individuals. In developed health systems these organizations interact and counter-balance one another's influence. Ideally, the outcome will be a balanced situation where all promote, and are responsible for, the effectiveness, quality and reputation of the health system. This balance is far from being reached in Nigeria, and one aim of any intervention should be to move health markets in this direction.

Considering this framework suggests three main dimensions in the relationship between healthcare providers and patients: trust, formal regulation and information flow. Crucial to understanding the role of these dimensions within the framework suggested here is an appreciation of the large number of stakeholders able to influence the success of the system. In the case of PMVs, key stakeholders include their trade associations, the bodies tasked with regulating the pharmaceutical sector, local government bodies that regulate small businesses and the local government health departments.

Trust is a key dimension in the relationships between providers and patients, its importance varying proportionally with the degree of asymmetry of information. Providers often adopt strategies to build trust and maintain a reputation for high expertise and ethics (Montagu, 2002, 2003; Mills *et al.*, 2002; Prata *et al.*, 2005).

Patients in Nigeria have shown a willingness to pay to access such providers. Trust and reputation are built on many factors, including brand recognition (e.g. franchise, accreditation or licensing) and perceived quality of services (e.g. staff qualifications and experience, equipment, cleanliness and courtesy). Less formal attributes may be important at the community level, such as a history of good behaviour, being an active member of the community, or family background.

Formal regulatory systems have often lagged far behind the rapid growth of health markets in developing countries. Many providers operate outside any legal framework. Barriers to effective regulation are often linked to a lack of government capacity for enforcement or the lack of incentives to enforce regulations (Ensor and Weinzieri, 2006).

Many health systems focus primarily on regulating the formal sector that meets the needs of the wealthier sections of the population, not the informal sector which serves the poor. To fill this gap, market actors have sometimes endeavoured to improve market functioning, for example by partnering with government to co-produce rules (Joshi and Moore, 2004; Peters and Muraleedharan, 2008). Others have created self-regulating organizations, for example social franchises. In Nigeria the activities of PMVs are regulated through government bodies, other professionals and PMV associations. The National Malaria Control Programme (NMCP) of the Federal Ministry of Health establishes standards and guidelines concerning the recommended first- and second-line drugs for the treatment of malaria, while a set of regulatory decisions revolving around which drugs are approved for use in a country are made by the food and drug regulatory agency. Moreover, the Pharmaceutical Association has laws on the types of medicines that could be dispensed and/or sold. These various policies and regulations are not necessarily in harmony. The PMV association engages in regulating its members with respect to what brands to sell and quality issues around expiry dates.

Another important aspect of the performance of health-related markets emphasized in the framework shown in Figure 7.1 is the flow of information. Some providers have access to organized education and training courses. Others simply learn on the job (through the PMV apprenticeship system, for example). Other key information sources are the traditional mass media (newspapers, television and radio) and new communication tools (e.g. mobile phones, the internet) that are used by commercial companies to advertise their medical and health-related products and by a wide variety of official and non-official, national and international, advocacy groups to communicate messages to providers, patients and the general population. For example, the PMV Association has recently been using its executive members to communicate with regulators and medicine supply chain managers and to reach consumers through advertising. This rapidly increasing volume of circulating information creates an urgent need for trusted knowledge brokers.

Perhaps the most important message from the framework shown in Figure 7.1 is the need to recognize just how many stakeholders influence the quantity and quality of health service provision and the complexity of the institutional context within which they function. Active stakeholder engagement not only is an essential aspect of health systems research but also is crucial for translating that research into sound public health policy and policy implementation.

Intervening in Nigerian informal markets: the politics of health market change

Empirical evidence suggests that PMVs play a central role in delivering malaria services. This makes them an important subject of research in understanding the dynamics of the health policy framework in Nigeria. Consider now the results of research focusing on the design of effective policies and programmes to combat malaria through private-sector partnerships. The research involved working alongside PMVs in regulatory partnerships involving government, civil society and the private sector to improve the services they provide in terms of both drug quality and of appropriate prescribing behaviour. The primary goal of FHS work in Nigeria was to contribute to national efforts to substantially increase the coverage of malaria control measures in response to the very high burden malaria places on poor people and the pressing need to expand access to effective and good-quality anti-malarial medicines. The initiative is described through the lens of the market framework outlined in Figure 7.1.

A policy analysis examining effective treatment of malaria was conducted nationally in 2006 to explore broader questions about problems in health system organization and possible solutions. Meanwhile, a detailed stakeholder analysis categorized key players, in terms both of intervention implementation and of strengthening the research–policy interface. On the basis of this analysis a mapping of knowledge and policy processes around malaria was developed. This mapping used a modified version of the framework proposed by Keeley and Scoones (2003) to understand policy processes in terms of interest groups, actor networks and performance of key institutions.

Scoping studies were conducted in three states selected to represent each of the major geographic and linguistic areas of Nigeria: Oyo State (south-west, Yoruba), Kaduna State (north-west, Hausa) and Enugu State (south-east, Igbo). Twelve rural and urban local government areas were used to better understand the market and the role played by PMVs in provision of anti-malarial drugs. These involved cross-sectional surveys of (110) PMVs and (113) households, supplemented by interviews with community leaders (54), PMV association officers (67) and government and health officials (31). Inventories were undertaken in PMV shops to assess the quantity and quality of available drugs. These studies indicated that PMVs were directly involved in the diagnosis and treatment of almost 40 per cent of fevers that were (rightly or wrongly) ascribed to malaria. They also sold most of the drugs that were used by around 25 per cent of cases where self-treatment was reported. Less than a quarter of all PMVs interviewed knew about the change in recommended malaria treatment from chloroquine to ACTs. Many still recommended and provided drugs whose efficacy is highly questionable: 92 per cent of shops had sulphadoxine-pyrimethamine in stock and 72 per cent chloroquine (both not recommended), whereas only 9 per cent had ACTs. More shops had monotherapy artesunates (32 per cent) than had ACTs, even though monotherapy is not recommended, owing to the risk of promoting drug resistance.

Drawing on the findings of the scoping studies, a series of interventions were designed to address the problems of inappropriate treatment and poor-quality drugs by reducing the opportunities for PMVs to knowingly misprescribe or supply substandard drugs. Each intervention involved a mix of components, including the following: increasing the effective control that PMV associations exercised over their members; ensuring an active role for communities in monitoring and regulation; the use of mobile phones to facilitate communication with and between PMVs; and promoting the introduction of simple new technologies for routine testing of anti-malarial drugs.

Increasing the effective control that PMV associations exercised over their members would entail strengthening the capacity of their members to deliver quality services. This would require use of participatory training processes to improve PMV performance through cascade training to enable them to improve the delivery of quality drugs for malaria, the provision of appropriate advice and referral of people who use their services. Such a training approach should appeal to conscience and the dangers inherent in putting customers in harm's way complemented by other ways of appealing to PMVs through better sourcing of drugs.

Ensuring an active role for communities in monitoring and regulation would increase community knowledge and engagement for monitoring drug quality. In this regard, compliance to quality drugs by PMVs would be monitored by local community watch groups (health task forces) composed of members of local organizations, civil society and experts who would adhere to agreed quality standards and use these to assess PMV shops' anti-malarial drug stocks and use the monitoring to determine which PMV shops could be franchised as 'Best Drug Shops'. Thus, the creation of effective regulatory partnerships could ensure the quality and affordability of drug supplies. Successful strategies for constructing more effective regulation increasingly involve partnerships between government, civil society organizations and the private sector. The relevant organizations need to include the regulatory arms of central and local government, professional and trade associations, large service provision organizations or civil society organizations, and consumer associations. Such regulatory partnerships could address unregulated markets in the distribution of low-quality and counterfeit drugs, thereby solving problems of safety, efficacy and cost. This intervention also included an element of 'branding' – with communities made aware of the partnerships between PMV associations and the University of Ibadan FHS team.

The use of mobile phones could increase PMVs' access to information on anti-malarial drugs, government policies, regulations and guidelines, and feedback from PMVs to government officials. This would facilitate communication with and between PMVs. Information and communications technology (ICT) using the MTN broadband TEXT can be used to empower government and PMV regulators, and empower communities by increasing the availability of information, knowledge on quality anti-malarial drugs and knowledge concerning government policies to PMVs. Using the MTN infrastructure and technological capability, the Malaria InfoText service to PMVs via SMS could enable Ministry of Health health workers to send information to and receive reports from PMVs concerning quality anti-malarial drugs being bought and sold, and the number of people who experienced drug side effects, or knew about government policies. This could help transform the development prospects of public and private organizations involved in this collaborative effort.

The promoting and introduction of simple new technologies for routine testing of anti-malarial drugs is critical. For example, smart equipment can be used to detect anti-malarial drugs that are counterfeit or sub-standard. The creative use of such technology would ensure that government and PMV regulators, and community drug monitors, have the tools they need to take advantage of opportunities and solve critical problems of counterfeit anti-malarial drugs both at the source of purchase and at points of distribution through PMV shops by testing samples of the drugs with a simple kit.

A large number of diverse stakeholders were identified, and the level of power and influence of each stakeholder profiled. The results were used by the team to guide the process of gaining approval, and where possible gaining active support, for the proposed research. This was seen as essential, given that the idea of strengthening malaria control interventions through PMVs has been strongly resisted in the past. The initial step was to convince the staff of National Coordinator for Malaria Control. This involved a series of consultations designed to move them from awareness, to interest, to serious consideration and finally to willingness to authorize pilot interventions. The principal argument in this case was that the intervention had the potential to provide a lasting political legacy in terms of making a substantial difference to malaria mortality in Nigeria. Similar advocacy processes were undertaken with the health minister, several directors of the Federal Ministry of Health (FMOH) (including the director responsible for pharmaceuticals), selected state commissioners of health and other stakeholders. To the extent possible, all these policy-makers were then engaged in further defining the research agenda.

All types of informants were concerned about the quality of the drugs. Although more government regulation was suggested by all parties, in this complex and highly unregulated market environment PMV associations were also identified by communities as potentially playing important roles in providing information, influencing PMV behaviour and procuring drugs. Interestingly, community involvement in drug regulation was viewed as highly desirable by the PMVs themselves (92 per cent).

A series of meetings at Abuja and Oyo State in 2007 and 2008 with all the relevant stakeholders were held to provide detailed presentations of the proposed interventions and to seek engagement on both refining their design and supporting implementation. Those attending these meetings included a range of national and local policy-makers, members of pharmaceutical associations, representatives of PMV associations, NGOs, drug (ACT) manufacturers and distributors, government regulators, and social entrepreneurs with a potential interest in innovative approaches to improving the supply chain of effective anti-malarial drugs. In addition, a major conference involving leading politicians from both legislative houses, health commissioners, and a range of national and international experts in health systems, innovators and social entrepreneurs was held in Abuja[1] on 12 and 13 January 2009 to debate and, where necessary, modify the intervention design.

Alongside this formal process, the research team exploited every opportunity to interact informally with key stakeholders in government, civil society, health service provider organizations, NGOs and other civil society organizations. The methods employed included attending public-health-related functions, sending congratulatory letters to new ministers, courtesy visits to policy-makers' offices when on other assignments, routine phone calls to update selected stakeholders on progress, and sending regular newsletters to ministers, commissioners, health and PHC directors and malaria managers at national and state levels.

Two FHS interventions by the Federal Ministry of Health's NMCP, comprising short- and longer-term training of PMVs in formal government institutions, and the creation of regulatory partnerships between government, PMV associations and community governance structures, were formally approved for programming. The formal adoption by senior policy-makers of interventions aimed at integrating PMVs into national malaria control interventions marks a significant departure from past policy. Funding support was requested and obtained by NMCP for pilot testing in seven malaria booster states, and implementation is ongoing.

The PMV associations are being strengthened through enhancing their capacity to deliver quality services (ACTs, counselling and referrals) consistent with government guidelines and best malaria treatment practices as well as contract-based performance in the area of training, supervision and internal monitoring. The study has helped reshape the national health policy and programme in favour of PMV integration into malaria control programs.

This work exemplifies how research institutions can use an innovative approach to influencing malaria policy and programmes through active engagement of stakeholders at all programme phases.

Conclusions

PMVs play a crucial role in providing health care for the rural poor in a country such as Nigeria, and especially in meeting the healthcare needs surrounding a major regional health problem such as malaria. Analysis must take into account the complex nature of the policy context in the country. The diagnosis and treatment of malaria provide a particular instance of this. PMVs often lack up-to-date drugs and have insufficient knowledge regarding prescription. Yet they also play a crucial role in tackling serious disease problems. This means that the performance of PMVs needs urgent improvement. The conceptual framework offered in this chapter provides a useful way to understand the important roles of both regulation and information flow in constructing useful market-based health interventions. However, a recurrent finding in this study, and in studies throughout this volume, is that it is essential to see healthcare provision as complex and as part of a complex wider context. The interventions that were studied in this project demonstrated the need to engage a range of stakeholders in dealing with matters of general concern, such as prescribing correct and in-date drugs, rather than merely looking to PMVs to get this right unilaterally. The most interesting intervention was in malaria treatment. With formal government involvement, as well as more participatory regulation regimes, it is believed that Nigeria can actively involve PMVs on the front line of reducing negative health effects of malaria. Moreover, doing so is likely to be more successful than the sorts of top-down criticizing methods that have been adopted in the past.

Notes

1   Online, available at: www.futurehealthsystems.org/nigeria/

References

Berman, P. and Rose, L. (1996) 'The role of private providers in maternal and child health and family planning services in developing countries', *Health Policy and Planning*, 11: 142–155

Bloom, G. (2001) 'Equity in health in unequal societies: meeting health needs in contexts of social change', *Health Policy*, 57 (3): 205–224

Bloom, G. (2004) 'Private provision in its institutional context: lessons from health', DFID Health Systems Resource Centre Issues Paper

Bloom, G. and Standing, H. (2001) 'Pluralism and marketisation in the health sector: meeting health needs in contexts of social change in low and middle-income countries', IDS Working Paper 136, Institute of Development Studies, Brighton

Bloom, G., Lloyd, R. and Standing, H. (2006) 'Rethinking future health systems', unpublished paper, Institute of Development Studies, Brighton

Brieger, W. R., Salami, K. K. and Oshiname, F. O. (2007) 'Perceptions of drug color among drug sellers and consumers in rural southwestern Nigeria', *Research in Social and Administrative Pharmacy*, 3 (3): 303–319

Commission on Health Research for Development (COHRED) (1990) *Health Research: Essential Link to Equity in Development*, Oxford University Press, New York

Das Gupta, M., Gauri, V. and Khemani, S. (2004) 'Decentralized delivery of primary health services in Nigeria: survey evidence from the states of Lagos and Kogi', Africa Region Human Development Working Paper Series 70, World Bank, Washington, DC

Ehiri, J. E., Oyo-Ita, A. E., Anyanwu, E. C., Meremikwu, M. M. and Ikpeme, M. B. (2005) 'Quality of child health services in primary health care facilities in south-east Nigeria', *Child: Care, Health and Development*, 31: 181–191

Elliot, D., Gibson, A. and Hitchins, R. (2008) 'Making markets work for the poor: rationale and practice', *Enterprise Development and Microfinance*, 19 (2): 101–119

Ensor, T. and Weinzieri, S. (2006) *A Review of Regulation in the Health Sector in Low and Middle Income Countries: Signposts to More Effective States*, Institute of Development Studies, Brighton

Global Forum for Health Research (1999) *The 10/90 Report on Health Research 1999*, Global Forum for Health Research, Geneva

Global Forum for Health Research (2000) *The 10/90 Report of Health Research 2000*, Global Forum for Health Research, Geneva

Hargreaves, S. (2002) 'Time to right the wrongs: improving basic health care in Nigeria', *Lancet*, 359 (9322): 2030–2035

Joshi, A. and Moore, M. (2004) 'Institutionalised co-production: unorthodox public service delivery in challenging environments', *Journal of Development Studies*, 40 (4): 31–39

Keeley, J. and Scoones, I. (2003) *Understanding Environmental Policy Processes: Cases from Africa*, Earthscan, London

Khemani, S. (2004) *Local Government Accountability for Service Delivery in Nigeria*, Development Research Group, World Bank, Washington, DC

Mackintosh, M. and Koivusalo, M. (2005) 'Health systems and commercialization: in search of good sense', in M. Mackintosh and M. Koivusalo (eds) *Commercialization of Health Care: Global and Local Dynamics and Policy Responses*, Palgrave Macmillan, Basingstoke, UK

Mills, A., Brugha, R., Hanson, K. and McPake, B. (2002) 'What can be done about the private health sector in low-income countries?', *Bulletin of the World Health Organization*, 80: 325–330

Montagu, D. (2002) 'Franchising of health services in low-income countries', *Health Policy and Planning*, 17 (2): 121–130

Montagu, D. (2003) 'Accreditation and other external quality assessment systems for health care', DFID Health Systems Resource Centre Working Paper, Department for International Development, London

National Population Commission of Nigeria (2008) *Nigeria Demographic and Health Survey*, ICF MACRO, Abuja

Peters, D. H. and Muraleedharan, V. R. (2008) 'Regulating India's health services: to what end? What future?', *Social Science and Medicine*, 66 (10): 2133–2144

Prata, N., Montagu, D. and Jefferys, E. (2005) 'Private sector, human resources and health franchising in Africa', *Bulletin of the World Health Organization*, 83 (4): 241–320

World Health Organization (2006) *Disease Control Priorities in Developing Countries*, 2nd ed., World Health Organization, Geneva

8   Yes, they can

Peer educators for diabetes in Cambodia

Maurits van Pelt, Henry Lucas, Chean Men, Ou Vun, MoPoTsyo and Wim Van Damme

Summary

It seems clear that Cambodia's health services cannot meet the enormous and rising needs of people with diabetes. Innovative approaches are required to mitigate the impact of the rising epidemic. One possible route is suggested by the concept of 'disruptive innovations', entailing a focus on models that, typically by exploring alternative input combinations, can deliver good low-cost products or services at a price that makes them accessible to the great majority of the population. One model that seems of particular interest in the treatment of diabetes is the 'facilitated user network', which uses the combined resources of a range of stakeholders – patients, their families, physicians, pharmaceutical suppliers and community workers – to construct supportive and mutually beneficial networks. Since 2005 the MoPoTsyo programme has been establishing diabetes 'peer educator networks' to detect and support diabetes patients. This study is based on analysis of routine monitoring data for 386 rural diabetes patients who have been enrolled in the programme for at least three months, and data from two assessments of a random sample of these patients, carried out in July 2008 and January 2009. After eighteen months, ten peer educators had found 474 diabetes patients, two-thirds of them previously unaware of their condition. The data on these patients indicate improvements in fasting and postprandial blood glucose, and blood pressure, even though half of them had not yet consulted a doctor. Their reported health expenditure appears much more affordable than that of most diabetes patients in Cambodia. In the absence of a massive government or international response to the unmet needs of Cambodians with diabetes, peer educator networks may play a useful role in mitigating the disease's negative impacts on the lives of sufferers by providing a low-cost but effective care structure despite the low-resource environment.

Introduction

There is increasing awareness of the widespread prevalence of chronic diseases and the consequent burdens on both populations and health services (Abegunde *et al.*, 2007). The WHO (2005) projects 388 million deaths from chronic diseases in the next ten years, the majority in the economically active age group and 80 per cent in low- and middle-income countries. The implications for these countries, many still struggling to cope with a high burden of infectious diseases and the AIDS pandemic, are extremely serious. Some appear to have decided that, given the perceived costs, providing adequate management of chronic illnesses is an unobtainable goal, at least over the short to medium term. In the absence of very substantial additional resources from the international community (Anderson, 2009), the prospects seem bleak, especially as the prevalence of many chronic illnesses appears to be rising inexorably, partly owing to increased longevity. There is a substantial risk that desperation will drive many people into the arms of unscrupulous individuals and organizations that will add to their financial burdens while failing to mitigate, or even worsening, their health problems. Innovative approaches are urgently needed.

This chapter focuses on one of the most important chronic diseases, diabetes (WHO, 2009). A recent *Lancet* article described it as 'now a global problem, equal in size to that of HIV/AIDS' (Lefèbvre and Silink, 2006). Much of that problem is hidden, with the majority of patients in poorer countries remaining undiagnosed. One group of these will, at least initially, be asymptomatic, while others will suffer on a daily basis from the multiple effects of hyperglycaemia, including nocturnal polyuria, relentless thirst, dry throat, permanent hunger, eczema, ulcers, dizziness and fatigue. Both undiagnosed and diagnosed patients will often receive inadequate or inappropriate care, adding the effects of medically induced hypoglycaemia to the panoply of potential symptoms. Healthcare providers frequently lack the training required to recognize the symptoms of poor glycaemic control. Health facilities often lack the resources to treat the causes. In consequence, a majority of patients suffer the early onset of long-term complications, often resulting in premature death. Yet much of this suffering can be delayed for years, and even prevented, if patients make suitable lifestyle changes and are given the opportunity to adhere to appropriate medication.

If neither public- nor private-sector health providers appear likely to deliver the required products and services to the great majority of diabetes sufferers, most of whom lack the resources typically needed to purchase quality care, it may be appropriate to explore more innovative approaches. A relatively recent conceptual framework for innovations research proposed by Bower and Christensen (1995) may provide clues as to the possible characteristics of such an approach. Bower and Christensen classified innovations into two categories: sustaining and disruptive. Most were seen as falling into the first category, offering improved quality or additional functionality. On the other hand, disruptive innovations typically offer simplicity, convenience and lower cost, possibly accompanied by a reduction in non-essential qualities, features or functions. One target audience for these new products or services would be those who had previously felt excluded by price or technical barriers to access.

A later paper (Christensen *et al.*, 2006) specifically discusses the potential implications of disruptive innovations in the social sectors. The core argument is that many service delivery organizations, both public and private, prioritize the provision of high-quality services even if this involves a serious trade-off in terms of the size of the population they are able to serve effectively. This situation may be motivated by the best of intentions. Those responsible for service provision are typically highly skilled and qualified individuals trained in, or at least with exposure to, health systems in countries that can afford to deliver high-quality services to large populations. As professionals, they cannot be blamed for aspiring to the 'best practice' standards established in such countries. They may react badly to what they would interpret as suggestions that their patients should be offered treatment that falls below those standards. On the other hand, as the paper argues, and very much in line with the situation relating to chronic illness discussed above, it is often inconceivable that sufficient resources will be made available to extend these best-practice services to all those in need.

The approach suggested in the paper is to promote organizations that engage in 'catalytic innovations', a sub-set of disruptive innovations focusing specifically on social change that offer 'good enough' alternatives to the underserved population. These organizations will rarely emerge from the ranks of established providers, given that they have 'resources, processes, partners, and business models designed to support the status quo'. They will rarely 'disrupt themselves' (Christensen *et al.*, 2006, p. 96). Again this argument seems plausible when applied to formal public and private healthcare providers in low-income countries. Hwang and Christensen (2008) explore this notion by considering the possible 'business models' that healthcare providers might adopt. For present purposes the most interesting of these is the 'facilitated user network'. This aims to provide opportunities for transactions between the members of a stakeholder network, with value deriving from the ease and quality of the transaction process. The article notes that such networks are already playing a limited role in the provision of health care. They are often focused on specific medical conditions, for example obesity, addiction and HIV/AIDS, where information exchange and social learning process are highly valued. In the next section we consider one such network that appears to demonstrate how positive change can be achieved for those affected by diabetes, even in one of the world's poorest countries.

Diabetes in Cambodia

Cambodia has a population of 13.4 million, 80 per cent living in rural areas. With a gross national income estimated at US$540 per capita for 2007 (World Bank, 2009), it faces severe problems in coping with both communicable and non-communicable diseases (Janssens *et al.*, 2007). Two epidemiological studies published in 2005 found over 250,000 people suffering from diabetes, two-thirds of them being unaware of their condition (King *et al.*, 2005). The dysfunctional diabetes healthcare environment is graphically illustrated by the title of a recent report, quoting from one sufferer: 'I wish I had AIDS' (Men *et al.*, 2012). That report describes how people consult multiple public and private providers in a costly but typically unsuccessful search for correct diagnosis and effective treatment. The appropriate medicine for most diabetes patients, an affordable oral generic drug, is available in private pharmacy outlets but extremely hard to locate among the plethora of medicines of varying price and unknown quality promoted by thousands of licensed and unlicensed pharmacies.

Diabetes is not yet part of the standard public health services package, and many qualified doctors are uncertain as to appropriate treatment. Without additional training and guidelines, the needs from over 80,000 diagnosed diabetics for basic health services cannot be met. With double that number unaware of their condition, alternative solutions must be considered to reduce the enormous gap between needs and response.

The MoPoTsyo Patient Information Centre (MoPoTsyo, 2009) is a Cambodian NGO using an innovative approach to diabetes diagnosis and management, based on the 'peer educator' (Paul *et al.*, 2007) and 'informed patient' (Kober and Van Damme, 2006; Henwood *et al.*, 2003) concepts. It aims to create empowered patient networks, each consisting of 500–1,000 registered members organized around a team of peer educators, to support the pursuit of affordable and trustworthy health care. It operates both internally – providing information on self-management, advice and counselling – and externally, mediating between those in need of care and a wide variety of public and private doctors, pharmacists and other service providers. A small salaried staff is employed to establish and support the semi-autonomous networks in building trust, identifying and training new peer educators and organizing themselves under a diabetes programme manager (DPM) appointed jointly by MoPoTsyo and the local health authority. MoPoTsyo also manages its own Revolving Drug Fund.

The peer educators, who receive six weeks' formal training, have themselves recently recovered from years of serious illness and gain the trust of their communities because they can relate personal experience of the effects of poor glycaemic control. After accreditation they qualify for basic equipment and supplies, based on reported activities, and are allowed to identify their home as a 'Patient Information Centre' for weekly patient gatherings and education sessions. Newly qualified educators will screen their community for diabetes. Initial screening is based on adults self-testing with urine strips. The educator counsels those with positive strips and confirms their result using a blood glucose meter. The critical levels are: fasting blood glucose (FBG) ≥126 mg (7.0 mmol) and/or postprandial blood glucose (PPBG) ≥180 mg (10.0 mmol). Peer educators are also trained to take a simple patient history using a form that records items including the measurements of FBG, PPBG, blood pressure (BP), urine glucose, weight and height. Screening will start within the peer educator's village and be extended over a period of one to two years to cover an area designated by MoPoTsyo in agreement with local health authorities.

Newly detected diabetics can only become registered members after approval from the DPM, who oversees all peer educators in the health district. The patient's record is then included in a database for follow-up by the peer educator, monthly reporting by the DPM to the health authorities and entry into the local network's own Khmer Open Source database. This is compatible with software used at the central level, where data can be aggregated and analysed.

New patients may attend six classes at the home of their peer educator. They are typically encouraged to stop smoking, become more physically active and improve or maintain weight. Peer educators discuss nutrition issues using the MoPoTsyo food pyramid, which is based on a glycaemic index (GI) of locally available food items (Figure 8.1). Every patient receives an A3-size poster to put on the wall.

The staple food of Cambodians is white rice, which is eaten three times each day. Unfortunately, the common variety is highly glycaemic (Seng, 2007), owing to machine polishing. One important piece of peer educator advice is to change from white rice to less polished or even to whole rice, mixed, for example, with mung beans (GI = 31) or other vegetables from the low-GI green area on the poster. All of these are also richer in protective vitamins and minerals than the

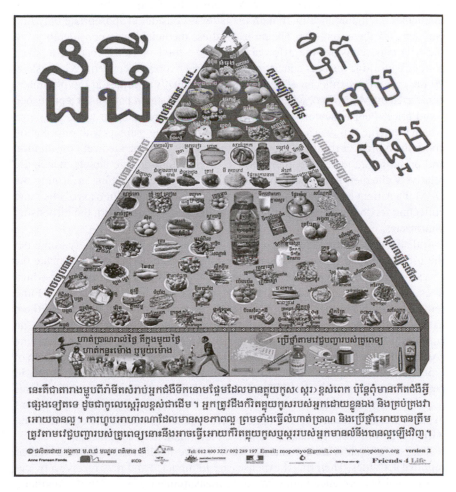

Figure 8.1 Glycaemic index food pyramid.

white rice. The use of beans as a staple is unheard of in rural Cambodia, where they are grown but eaten as a dessert, boiled in sugar water.

Patients are provided with urine glucose strips each month. They are encouraged to use these within three hours of eating to detect after-meal glucose peaks. This relatively simple self-testing procedure is easily learned and reasonably reliable, provided that kidney function has not deteriorated. Patients are also asked to perform a twenty-four-hour urine test twice a month. All test results are recorded in their self-management book.

If lifestyle changes produce insufficient results within a few months, or sooner if warranted by the patient's condition, peer educators assist patients to obtain an appointment with a specially trained medical doctor (MD). In practice, they function as gatekeepers for such visits. This MD is contracted by MoPoTsyo to hold consultations at the local public hospital once per week to initiate or change medical treatments for diabetics. The MD prescribes from a limited list of twenty medicines, including insulin, though the latter is considered appropriate only in 5 per cent of diabetes patients. The prices of these medicines vary considerably and the MD must consider the affordability of the total monthly cost for a given patient, consulting the peer educator if that patient expresses concern. When asked, 90 per cent of patients can afford to buy prescribed medicines at the pharmacy contracted by MoPoTsyo, where they are sold to registered patients at a published fixed price. Peer educators are instructed *never* to prescribe or advise patients which medicine to buy. Their role is limited to providing patients with information about the typical cost ranges they can expect if they go for medical consultation and prescription; to show patients how to divide high-dosage tablets, which are relatively cheaper, into pieces that meet their daily requirements; informing the DPM if a patient has a prescription for a drug that is not on MoPoTsyo's list; and collecting feedback from the patients about their experiences with the dispensing pharmacies.

Initially, consultation costs were met by MoPoTsyo's Health Equity Fund, but the use of the fund for this purpose is no longer common practice. To make the service financially sustainable, the patients have agreed to pay a user fee, which does not include the prescribed routine medication. The Health Equity Fund remains available to the very poor, about 10 per cent of patients, and assists them to pay for the cheapest available prescription options. There is, for example, no support to help a patient buy a more expensive angiotensin-converting enzyme (ACE) inhibitor instead of a cheaper beta blocker. A relatively large proportion of type 2 diabetics requiring insulin receive this assistance, which covers up to 50 per cent of their monthly costs. The assistance is possible because so few patients require insulin and its provision in these cases is seen as meeting the expectations of the wider community. Every opportunity is taken to reduce the cost of living with diabetes in order to make the intervention financially sustainable.

The peer educators are not salaried. They receive small incentives based on their reported activities. Their travel expenses are reimbursed and they receive a twice-yearly total performance bonus based on measurement of some thirty, regularly changing, outcomes on a random sample of nineteen of their patients. The July

2008 assessment bonuses varied in size from US$29 to US$72, paid to seven peer educators who had more than 300 patients to follow up.

Data

This study is based on analysis of:

*   Routine registration and follow-up data collected between 1 July 2007 and 31 December 2008 by peer educators on 386 rural diabetes mellitus patients enrolled in MoPoTsyo for at least three months, including FBG, PPBG, urine glucose, BP and body weight.
*   Data from two assessments carried out by trained health workers in July 2008 and January 2009 of 133 and 152 randomly sampled patients respectively, including HbA1c, body weight, reported health-related expenditure, data related to self-management knowledge and skills, and patient opinions as to peer educators and care. The blood samples were analysed at the Diabetes Service of National Kossamak Hospital to assess the HbA1c (glycated haemoglobin), using a Biorad D-10 Hemoglobin A1c testing system.
*   Health expenditure data for households with a patient with diabetes are extracted from a household survey in rural Cambodia conducted by the Center for Advanced Study as part of the POVILL Consortium (POVILL, 2009).

Findings

Screening, detection and retention of diabetics

Over the eighteen months ending 31 December 2008, peer educators reached more than 80 per cent of adults among the district population, with 53,839 using a urine glucose strip after a meal. Of those testing positive, 474 were confirmed as diabetic following a further blood glucose test and all registered with MoPoTsyo. Sixty-seven per cent had previously been unaware of the cause of their ill health. As can be seen in Figure 8.2, the total number of members grew steadily even though 11 per cent of registered patients departed (3 per cent dying, 4 per cent leaving the area and 4 per cent losing interest).

Lifestyle counselling and self-monitoring

In the second assessment, 41 per cent of patients claimed that they engaged in strenuous physical labour or exercise for more than three hours per week. Almost all (94 per cent) of the remainder indicated that they knew that they should do more, and 87 per cent of patients reported that their activity level had increased after entering the programme. Around 84 per cent of patients said that they had reduced the quantity of white rice in their diet. Sixty-three per cent had a body mass index (BMI) that had either remained in the normal range (18.5–23.0) or improved since enrolment. Among those whose BMI value had worsened, 85 per

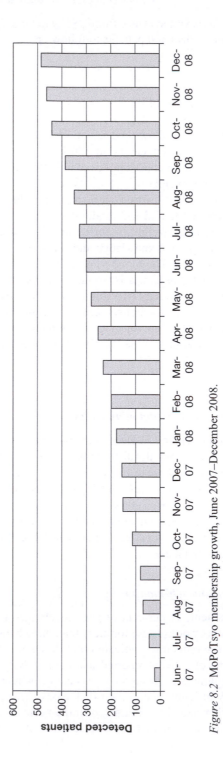

Figure 8.2 MoPoTsyo membership growth, June 2007–December 2008.

cent had gained weight. Overall, 46 per cent were overweight (BMI >23.0) and 11 per cent obese (BMI >27.5), while 14 per cent had a BMI ≤18.5. Peer education on this issue has not proved entirely straightforward. Almost a quarter of those concerned did not accept the suggested need to adjust their weight.

Review of patient self-management books indicated that 71 per cent had recorded more than two urine glucose results over the previous month. This figure was depressed by the 5 per cent rate in one new peer educator area, while the other seven had rates of 80 per cent or more. The complicated 24-hour urine test proved more problematic, with just over 40 per cent of patients being able to correctly describe the procedure.

Medical consultations, prescriptions and reported health expenditure

As is indicated in Figure 8.3, 44 per cent of patients have not yet seen a physician, while 2 per cent have had 13 or more visits. Overall, the average number of consultations per patients was 2, but this varied substantially (from 0.67 to 3.49) between peer educators.

Some 55 per cent of patients have thus far been put on prescription drugs at some point. Table 8.1 provides a detailed breakdown of the drugs prescribed by consultation sequence. This indicates that glibenclamide is prescribed for 70 per cent of patients attending an initial consultation, while insulin is prescribed for just 2 per cent. After the second consultation, the glibenclamide frequency gradually increases to a maximum of 88 per cent at the time of the fourth consultation, but

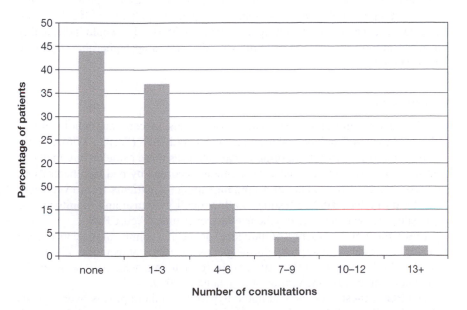

Figure 8.3 Percentage of patients receiving MD consultations, June 2008–December 2008.

Table 8.1 Content of prescriptions at the first and second consultations

Consultation	First	Second
Number of prescriptions	263	166
Aspirin 300mg	71%	73%
Glibenclamide 5mg	70%	77%
Metformin HCl 500mg	56%	68%
Vitamin B	46%	44%
Atenolol 100mg	44%	39%
Amitriptyline 25mg	29%	30%
Paracetamol 500mg	26%	25%
Captopril 25mg	19%	19%
Hydrochlorothiazide 50mg	13%	22%
Furosemide 40mg	8%	7%
Insulin-NPH 10ml	2%	1%
Insulin-Lantus 3ml	0%	1%

prescription of insulin remains a rare event. In fact, the prescription profile does not change much, despite frequent consultations. This is partly because it reflects a series of compromises between medical needs and cost affordability for individual patients.

In the January 2009 assessment, patients reported average health-related expenditure of US$3.19 per month, varying from US$1.13 to US$5.53 across different peer educators. Unpublished data from a recent household survey (Lucas *et al.*, 2008) indicate that forty rural Cambodians reporting diabetes had spent an average of US$52.06 per month. Only four reported expenditures below US$3.41, while half paid more than US$13.9 and eight more than US$61. This would indicate that for most Cambodians the cost of living with diabetes is far higher than for those within MoPoTsyo.

Glucose control

Initial screening measures FBG and PPBG levels in capillary whole blood, following the cut-off points established in WHO guidelines (WHO, 2006). Mainly on cost grounds, routine monitoring of patients uses these same testing methods complemented by urine glucose measurements recorded by patients themselves. The six-monthly assessments of a random sample of patients from every peer educator do include HbA1c testing to allow quality control and monitoring of aggregate glucose control across the network over time (Figure 8.4).

Measurement of the progress of individual or specific cohorts of patients is done by using BG tests and interpreting urine glucose results. For example, Figure 8.5 provides 2008 quarterly mean BG levels for patients who had been in the programme for at least one year prior to 1 January 2009.

The FBG of most patients with initial hyperglycaemia improves over time, as indicated by Figure 8.6, which shows quarterly measurements for all those with FBG >10 mmol in quarter 4, 2007.

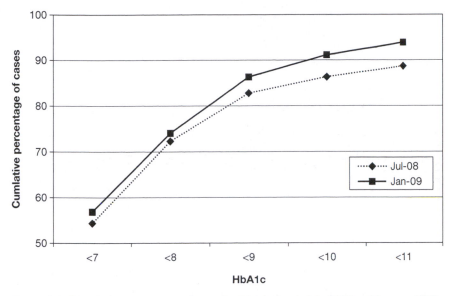

Figure 8.4 Cumulative percentage of cases by HbA1c level, July 2008 and January 2009.

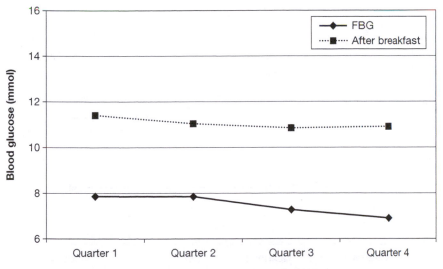

Figure 8.5 Quarterly means for routine BG values (mmol), 2008.

Blood pressure

High blood pressure increases the chance of developing serious complications. The peer educators will probe the patient for action if a patient's resting BP is greater than 130/80. Figure 8.7 shows quarterly average systolic and diastolic blood pressure readings for patients who had been in the programme for at least one year.

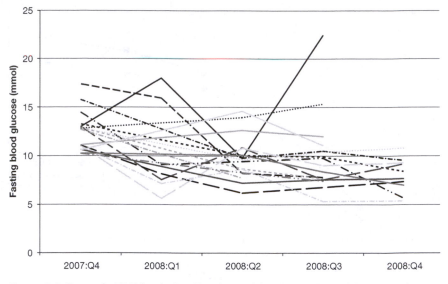

Figure 8.6 Quarterly FBG levels for all patients with values >10 mmol in quarter 4, 2007.

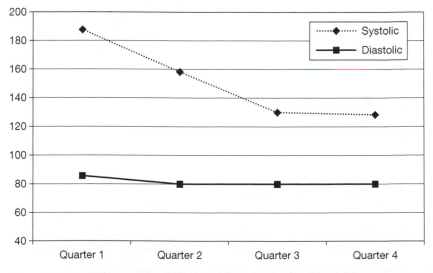

Figure 8.7 Quarterly means for systolic and diastolic blood pressure (mmHg), 2008.

Discussion

The experience with peer educators for diabetes in Cambodia shows that it is possible to detect many diabetics in the community, to organize them in peer support networks and support them towards lifestyle changes and self-management. The documented short-term improvements in blood glucose control and in blood pressure are encouraging, as well as the low number of medical consultations deemed necessary, the affordable level of health expenditures and the low drop-out rates. However, the rallying cry in the title of the chapter is not intended to proclaim a breakthrough in technical diabetes care but rather to indicate the potential for peer educator networks to complement professional caregivers, especially where those are scarce, expensive or less effective. The sobering fact is that for the foreseeable future, a great majority of those with diabetes in developing countries will not have access to trained health professionals. The limited number of practitioners will typically have other priorities than implementing the International Diabetes Federation guidelines (IDF Clinical Guidelines Task Force, 2005) on minimal levels of care.

The MoPoTsyo strategy appears to tap into a new pool of human health resources by involving recovered patients in undertaking rudimentary healthcare tasks for their fellow community members. They have the great advantage of local credibility. This enables them, as indicated earlier in the chapter, to persuade most community members to undertake preliminary self-testing, an extremely valuable outcome given that two-thirds of those identified were previously unaware of their condition. They can be an effective local source of information and motivation for people without alternatives, helping them to come to terms with both lifestyle changes and their longer-term prospects. Organizing the peer educators into a local network not only created a structure with a public presence but allowed mediated interaction with key professionals and organizations, including medical doctors, pharmacists and drug wholesalers.

A recent special issue of *Social Science and Medicine* (Bloom *et al.*, 2008) argued for a new approach to health systems that accepted the reality that a 'multiplicity of actors and institutions' were now involved in healthcare production. Progress depended on finding innovative ways of working within that context – not in denying or regretting it. The MoPoTsyo approach can be seen as one such innovation, with peer educators as a new form of community health worker (Standing *et al.*, 2008) adapted to the special needs of patients with a lifelong chronic disease, for whom self-management and peer support seem especially valuable.

The innovation raises questions that require further study. How can the peer educator networks best complement diabetes services where those are available? How should the approach be adapted to address multiple chronic diseases? The vertical national programmes for TB and HIV/AIDS already work with peer educators. Would it be sensible for multiple peer educators to work in the same community or even follow the same patient? Should peer educators actually 'peer-educate' on a disease or even a co-morbidity that they have not experienced themselves?

Arguably, there seems to be inherent merit in organizing and supporting diabetic patients towards lifestyle changes and self-management. The relation that the networks develop with professional healthcare systems will depend most of all on local realities and on locally negotiated arrangements. Inevitably, in a country like Cambodia the challenge posed by diabetes is so huge and the current health system so under-resourced that peer educators may have to play a larger role. They will need support in doing so, not as an easy or quick fix but as a labour-intensive strategy to build capacity at the level where it is most needed and immediately relevant.

The above discussion was introduced by reference to the concept of disruptive innovation. It may finally be worth reflecting on a related, and to some extent overlapping, concept, that of 'reverse innovation' (Immelt *et al.*, 2009). This refers to innovations that are likely to be first adopted in less developed countries or regions. Such innovations may well be disruptive if the primary reason for their development outside more highly developed areas is to appeal to a low-income population in a market that is primarily driven by price. However, it is suggested that once a low-cost basic product or service is available and shown to be of reasonable quality, it may well prove attractive to richer populations, or at least to those responsible for providing services to those populations. This process would be enhanced if the quality of the service could be gradually increased while maintaining the low price. Could networks such as that described above make a serious contribution to chronic care in highly developed nations? That may depend on the extent to which economic constraints lead to increased pressure on established health organizations, with both disruptive and reverse innovations potentially threatening existing practices and institutional arrangements.

References

Abegunde, D.O., Mathers, C. D., Adam, T., Ortegun, M. and Strong, K. (2007) 'The burden and costs of chronic diseases in low-income and middle-income countries', *Lancet*, 370: 1929–1938

Anderson, G. (2009) 'Missing in action: international aid agencies in poor countries to fight chronic disease', *Health Affairs*, 28: 202–205

Bloom, G., Standing, H. and Lloyd, R. (2008) 'Markets, information asymmetry and health care: towards new social contracts', *Social Science and Medicine*, 66 (10): 2067–2075

Bower, J. L. and Christensen, C. M. (1995) 'Disruptive technologies: catching the wave', *Harvard Business Review*, January–February: 43–53

Christensen, C. M., Baumann, H., Ruggles, R. and Sadtler, T. M. (2006) 'Disruptive innovation for social change', *Harvard Business Review*, December

Henwood, F., Wyatt, S., Hart, A., and Smith, J. (2003) '"Ignorance is bliss sometimes": constraints on the emergence of the "informed patient" in the changing landscapes of health information', *Sociology of Health and Illness*, 25 (6): 589–607

Hwang, J. and Christensen, C. M. (2008) 'Disruptive innovation in health care delivery: a framework for business-model innovation', *Health Affairs*, 27 (5): 1329–1335

IDF Clinical Guidelines Task Force (2005) *Global Guideline for Type 2 Diabetes*, International Diabetes Federation, Brussels

Immelt, J. R., Govindarajan, V. and Trimble, C. (2009) 'Reverse innovation: how GE is disrupting itself', *Harvard Business Review*, October

Janssens, B., Van Damme, W., Raleigh, B., Gupta, J., Khem, S., Soy, T. K., Vun, M. and Sachariah, R. (2007) 'Offering integrated care for HIV/AIDS, diabetes and hypertension within chronic disease clinics in Cambodia', *Bulletin of the World Health Organization*, 85 (11): 880–885

King, H., Keuky, L., Seng, S., Touch, K., Roglic, G. and Pinget, M. (2005) 'Diabetes and associated disorders in Cambodia: two epidemiological studies', *Lancet*, 366: 1633–1639

Kober, K. and Van Damme, W. (2006) *Expert Patients and AIDS Care: A Literature Review on Expert Patient Programmes in High-Income Countries, and an Exploration of Their Relevance for HIV/AIDS Care in Low-Income Countries with Severe Human Resource Shortages*, Institute of Tropical Medicine, Antwerp and Berlin

Lefèbvre, P. and Silink, M. (2006) 'Diabetes fights for recognition', *Lancet*, 368: 1625

Lucas, H., Ding, S. and Bloom, G. (2008) 'What do we mean by "major illness"? The need for new approaches to research on the impact of ill-health on poverty', in B. Meessen, X. Pei, B. Criel and G. Bloom (eds) *Health and Social Protection: Experiences from Cambodia, China and LaoDPR*, ITGPress, Antwerp

Men, C., Meessen, B., van Pelt, M., Van Damme, W. and Lucas, H. (2012) '"I wish I had AIDS": qualitative study on health care access among HIV/AIDS and diabetic patients in Cambodia', *Culture and Society*, 1 (2)

MoPoTsyo Patient Information Centre (2009) website, available at: www.MoPoTsyo.org (accessed 10 January 2009)

Paul, G., Smith, S. M., Whitford, D., O'Kelly, F. and O'Dowd, T. (2007) 'Development of a complex intervention to test the effectiveness of peer support in type 2 diabetes', *BMC Health Services Research*, 7: 136–146

POVILL Consortium (2009) 'Protecting the rural poor against the economic challenge of major illness: a challenge for Asian transitional economies'. Online, available at: www.ist-world.org/ProjectDetails.aspx?ProjectId=13e07d01d1a54f5cb1fe0975bcd63a39&SourceDatabaseId=7cff9226e582440894200b751bab883f (accessed 9 February 2009)

Seng, S. (2007) 'Studying changes in glycaemic index of white rice according to how it is prepared'. Unpublished, available at: www.mopotsyo.org/20070730GI-final.pdf (accessed 5 February 2009)

Standing, H., Mushtaque, A. and Chowdhury, R. (2008) 'Producing effective knowledge agents in a pluralistic environment: what future for community health workers?', *Social Science and Medicine*, 66: 2096–2107

WHO (2005) *Preventing Chronic Disease: A Vital Investment*, World Health Organization, Geneva

WHO (2006) *Definition and Diagnosis of Diabetes Mellitus and Intermediate Hyperglycaemia*, Report of a WHO/IDF Consultation, World Health Organization, Geneva

WHO (2009) Diabetes programme. Online, available at: www.who.int/diabetes/facts/world_figures/en/index.html (accessed 10 January 2009)

World Bank (2009) World Development Indicators. Online, available at: http://go.worldbank.org/1SF48T40L0 (accessed 5 February 2009)

9 Evidence of the effects of market-based innovations and international initiatives to improve the performance of private providers

Claire Champion, Gerald Bloom and David H. Peters

Introduction

This chapter identifies market-based innovations and international initiatives shown to affect the performance of providers in meeting the needs of the poor and likely to have a major impact on health-related markets in the future. We faced major challenges in putting this information together. There are no definitive inventories of innovations or initiatives in health-related markets and there is relatively little scientific literature on the performance of private providers, particularly in informal markets. Much activity takes place outside a formal regulatory structure and is not subject to reporting requirements. Some of the populous countries are experiencing very rapid increases in the demand for goods and services and in the growth of local and international companies. It is a challenge to obtain information on companies in these countries and the strategies they are formulating to capture market shares. Many of the international initiatives are still at a pilot stage and very little information is available about their performance. Many studies do not have strong study designs, limiting the ability to interpret what works. Finally, it is very challenging to generalize about a wide spectrum of low- and middle-income countries that differ in almost every way, and about organizations with diverse missions, forms and funding sources that are implementing mechanisms and performing at different levels of care from community-based services to specialty hospital care. We were, however, able to identify common trends and draw preliminary lessons about key factors of performance. One common theme is the importance of incentives and accountabilities within organizations and between organizations and other actors in the market system.

Review of innovations

The organized sector

This subsection presents the findings of an inventory of innovations in the organized sector compiled by Claire Champion. It is largely based on interviews with key stakeholders over a number of years, supplemented with information from the websites of umbrella and implementing organizations.[1] Although she made every effort to be comprehensive, the inventory is biased in favor of interventions supported by donor agencies, those inspired by developed country experiences and imported by developing markets, and models initiated by well-established local organizations. Those undertaken by private companies and local actors are likely to be greatly under-represented. It is difficult to assess the relative importance of these different sources of institutional innovation.

The models presented in the inventory show common trends but they differ greatly in their missions, forms, funding sources and implementing mechanisms. We have tried to avoid the use of ideal-type categorizations, such as 'social franchising', adapted from advanced market economies, to describe an organizational arrangement in a very different context.

Innovations are taking place at all levels of care from community-based services[2] to specialty hospital care.[3] Some organizations focus on one level of care and refer patients to the public or private sectors. Others provide two or more levels of care with referral mechanisms.[4] These organizations cover a large spectrum of health services. Some address family planning or HIV/AIDS and TB needs, whereas others offer a broader approach such as meeting essential drugs needs. Innovations have also taken place in the laboratories and diagnostic services industry.[5]

The self-defined missions of organizations include non-profit, commercial and faith-based ones. Whereas the commercial for-profit model has a clear mandate for financial sustainability, non-profit status is not a clear indication of the mission or financial objectives of the organization. Some non-profit organizations have introduced an up-front objective to reach financial sustainability within the first few years of their activities, and others anticipate a need for subsidies for a very long time.[6] We identified five categories of funding, including equity, loans or micro-credit, endowment set up by donors, donors' grants and others. More details are provided in Table 9.1. Little is known about the degree to which different sources of finance affect the values and management of an organization.

There is a proliferation of bottom-up and commercial models in Asia. This is most likely due to the better entrepreneurship environment of the region as well as growing and recognized market opportunities. Africa seems to favor imported models such as franchises, as well as faith-based initiatives. However, this is not the case in all countries (e.g. Nigeria or South Africa). In addition, the inventory might not provide adequate representation of volume and types of initiatives per country and per continent. One noticeable trend, however, is that most for-profit ventures target an urban market.[7] A few recent initiatives have tried to target rural areas with full cost recovery targets,[8] but many recognize the challenge of working in rural areas because of lower population density and the higher cost of monitoring and controlling quality.

Innovations have a number of sources. Some are the results of local or international entrepreneurs spotting a commercial and social opportunity.[9] Existing companies have also looked into opportunities to extend their outreach to

Table 9.1 Sources of funding

Category of funding	Sources	Examples
Equity	• Commercial investors and banks • International investors (e.g. IFC and Acumen Fund) • Parent company	• LifeSpring hospital is a joint venture between Acumen Fund and Hindustan Latex Ltd, a public-sector company. • Scojo Foundation has been initially funded by Scojo Inc.
Loans and micro-credit	• Banks • Micro-credit organizations	• In the case of franchises, franchisors have generally partnered with micro-finance organizations to provide start-up loans to franchisees. CFWshops initiated a partnership with a micro-finance organization to grant $2,000 loans to nurses to enable them to rehabilitate their clinic according to the franchise's standards, attend and pay for the franchise trainings and buy stock of products for the first month. The franchisor guarantees the loan.
Endowment fund	• International donors	• USAID provided an endowment fund of $5 million dollars to ProSalud in 1997 (Cuellar *et al.*, 2000). The objective was to help the organization reach financial sustainability through scale without rising prices.
Grants	• International donors (e.g. USAID, the Bill and Melinda Gates Foundation, DFID, KFW and GTZ)	• The Gateses funded MSH Seam project supported the development of the ADDO Shops network and the CareShops franchise.[a] • The USAID PSP-One Project provides, among other projects, technical assistance to Total Health Trust in Nigeria to help the entity in its scaling process.[b] • USAID also funded an institutional capacity-building project (the Capacity Project) to support faith-based organizations.[c]
Other donations	• National governments • Other organizations	• The government of Bolivia provided free lands to build the ProSalud new clinics and hospitals (Cuellar *et al.*, 2000).

Notes
a   www.msh.org/seam
b   www.psp-one.com
c   www.psp-one.com

lower-income populations and create their own distribution systems.[10] Some health franchising models are a direct extension of previous social marketing activities in which a franchising agreement has been signed with distribution outlets to increase incentives for quality.[11] Other initiatives are the result of independent health providers looking at improving their work's efficiency and quality and deciding to create their own association or network.[12] Lastly, the faith-based organizations provide services out of their religious mandate and fill needs unmet by the public sector.

We identified three types of quality control mechanism: a mix of management incentives and strict monitoring, a contractual approach with a branded franchise, and an accreditation mechanism. In the accreditation model, quality control is outsourced to the local authority,[13] while franchises internalize quality control. Franchisees are motivated to abide by the requirements of the franchise so that they can remain part of the franchise and benefit from its advantages (e.g. brand recognition, quality and affordable drugs, training, and professional network). In some franchises, franchisees are allowed to provide additional services that do not fall under the franchise rules,[14] while in others the franchisees are only authorized to provide a limited list of services and products.[15] Other organizations use a mix of management incentives and strict monitoring and quality control activities. They set up standardized procedures and guidelines and create a strong corporate culture for quality improvement.[16]

Brand and reputation are generally of prime importance. The asymmetry of information between the providers and their patients creates the need for patients to base their decision on reputation and signs they can recognize. Many of the organizations have developed large marketing and community outreach activities in order to enhance trust between the patients and the organization.[17]

All innovations claim to have a very strong patient-centered approach and to have defined their business model on the basis of this approach in order to meet patients' need for quality interaction, tailored information and organizational flexibility. The great majority of innovations position their products or services on principles such as staff being courteous and friendly, health workers and drugs being available, continuity of care, a clean environment, and flexible evening and weekend hours and/or a guarantee of confidentiality.[18] Health care, as is the case for many other services that target the poor in developing countries, is characterized by a high level of interactions and interpersonal relationships. Innovations also aim at lowering the hidden costs associated with public healthcare services. Hidden costs relate to transaction and accessibility costs. Transaction costs include waiting time, drugs stock-out and the necessity to buy the drugs in the market anyway, lack of continuity of care, and the need to see many people in many different places or overwhelming paperwork and forms to fill to process. Accessibility costs include transportation time and costs, reduced opening hours or opportunity costs of not being at work. Those costs are incurred even if public health care is provided for free and present a barrier as high as, if not higher than, the consultation or drug fees. Innovations are systematically targeting those costs as a strategy to increase their competitiveness to the public sector.[19]

There is a lot of evidence of rapid institutional development in the pharmaceutical sector. Both China and India have large firms that are becoming important global suppliers of pharmaceutical products. The development of the wholesale and retail markets has been slower, and there are serious problems with cost and quality in both countries. One important development in India has been the rapid creation of retail pharmacy chains. A review for this report identified seven that have announced plans to establish 8,000 shops over the next few years. Most shops are in urban areas, but there are also plans to establish low-cost rural pharmacies. These chains have involved a number of different actors, including a large pharmaceutical manufacturer, a US-based pharmacy franchise, a large hospital chain and a network of rural shops. It is difficult to predict the ultimate alignments that might emerge between these actors, or how these will affect the quality of drugs supplied and the kind of advice provided on prescriptions. This raises important challenges concerning regulation and consumer information. It is conceivable that India will become an important source of institutional innovation in retail pharmacy.

Informal markets

This subsection summarizes the types of interventions found in a systematic review of the literature on interventions to improve health services from informal providers of health-related goods and services in low- and middle-income countries (Shah *et al.*, 2010). The rationale for the review was the observation that informal providers are a major source of primary care services globally and represent a neglected opportunity for providing quality health services to people living in low- and middle-income countries. Of the seventy studies that were identified through systematic searching, only twenty-four (34 percent) of them were designed with comparisons and observations made at two points in time or more so that the size of the effect of the intervention could be estimated. A wide variety of interventions were involved, with most of them involving supply-side management strategies intending to improve performance of the informal providers. More than three-quarters of the interventions involved training of informal providers, about one-third involved the provision of supply (such as birthing kits) and one-quarter provided job aides to improve diagnosis and treatment. There were a smaller number of interventions involving organizational innovation (e.g. franchising and creation of new organizations), financial incentives and regulatory interventions. There was also some clustering in the content areas of the interventions. The control of infectious diseases, including HIV, was the most common medical area involved (51 percent of studies), followed by reproductive health issues (44 percent of studies) and child health (26 percent of studies).

Evidence of the performance of innovations

Organized markets

Many innovations are still at a pilot stage. There is still very little information available on their performance. We reviewed evidence in peer-reviewed journals and gray literature identified through a search of PubMed, Popline and Google and visits to websites of umbrella organizations. Most reports are of case studies. Although they do not always provide formal and rigorous evaluations, case studies are an important source of information. We found a few general reviews of evidence on private for-profit sector interventions (HLSP Institute, 2004; Mills *et al.*, 2002; Patouillard *et al.*, 2007; Prata *et al.*, 2005). Other reviews focus on family planning (WHO, 2007; Peters *et al.*, 2004; PSP-One, 2006), accreditation and certification (Shawn, 2001), or on faith-based organizations (Reinikka and Svensson, 2003). Koehlmoos *et al.* (2009) conducted a Cochrane review of the effect of social franchising on access to and quality of health services in low- and middle-income countries and did not find any eligible study for inclusion. All these reviews mention the lack of systematic evidence on impact and the need for rigorous evaluations. Most studies concern highly subsidized models such as social franchises and models that focus on family planning and reproductive health services. Three main outcomes have been studied: client satisfaction, quality of services and access by the poor. The first has been assessed in the majority of the studies, but very few studies measure quality of services and access to the poor. We could not find any evaluation on population health outcome or on the macroeconomic impact of those innovations.

Franchising models have been found to increase clients' satisfaction and perception of quality, and have tended to lead to an increase in service use (Agha *et al.*, 2007; PSI, 2007; Plautz *et al.*, 2003; Stephenson *et al.*, 2004). The few studies that explored objective measures of quality had mixed results. Impact varies within the same organization, with important differences between locations and across services and chosen criteria to measure quality (PSI, 2007; Prata *et al.*, 2005). When Stephenson and colleagues (2004) assessed family franchises in India (Janani), Pakistan (Greenstar and Green Key) and Ethiopia (Biruh Tesfa, Ray of Hope), they found an increased volume of services but did not find any association with reproductive health outcome.

The very few studies that assess access by the poor show mixed results. A study by Montagu *et al.* (2005) in Kenya concluded that the K-MET network did not increase inequalities in access to health services in rural areas. Hennink and Clements (2004) showed that even if the services are offered in poor neighborhoods in Pakistan, users of the services are not the urban poor themselves but select sub-groups of the local population. Several papers outline the trade-off between serving the poor, offering quality services and making a profit (PSP-One, 2006). Patouillard and colleagues (2007) emphasize the need to assess the impact of interventions on the poor.

A review of accreditation schemes by Shawn (2001) found that they seem to work well in middle- and high-income countries but have shown few results in low-income countries. However, an evaluation of a network of accredited drug-dispensing outlets in Tanzania showed a major decrease in the availability of unregistered drugs in the intervention group, suggesting an increase in drug quality (Sigonda-Ndomondo *et al.*, 2003).

Another strategy that builds on existing structures has been the efforts by associations of nurses or midwives in Central and Eastern Africa to enable their members to practice privately. In many of these countries the nurses have established a powerful position in the public sector but have been excluded from private practice. More recently, these restrictions have been removed, but institutional arrangements to support their establishment of a practice and build their reputations are not well developed (Rolfe *et al.*, 2008).

Another source of legitimacy in many countries is the many different faith communities. Reinikka and Svensson (2003) found that faith-based hospitals provided higher-quality health services at a lower cost in Uganda. Studies have demonstrated the great importance of networks associated with a religious denomination in building trust in many parts of Africa. A variety of health-related initiatives have built on this social capital. One example is the community health insurance schemes that have been linked to a church hospital or the church hierarchy. Another is the reputation that church hospitals tend to have for competence and ethical behavior. In fact, studies have shown a considerable amount of variation in the performance of different church hospitals (Tibandebage and Mackintosh, 2005), depending on local relationships. Nonetheless, it would appear that the identification of a hospital with a well-known religious denomination tends to enhance its reputation (Leonard, 2002).

Informal markets

Just over half (56 percent) of all the outcomes evaluated by studies testing interventions by informal providers were positive, suggesting that many of the interventions did not have much effect. As is shown in Table 9.2, which includes analysis from only the strongest study designs, there were many different types of interventions that were tested. The interventions most likely to succeed included social marketing, creating referral systems and training of trainers. Training by itself was the least successful approach (21 percent). These findings suggest that training plays a supplementary approach that should be included as part of other interventions.

It was also found that the greater the number of interventions, the more likely it was that positive outcomes would be found (Table 9.3). This suggests that having complementary interventions is important when working with informal providers, or that those informal providers that are able to handle more interventions are more likely to succeed.

Clearly, there is interest in testing strategies to improve health services from informal private providers in developing countries. The strategies that seem to be most successful are those that build on changing the market conditions, incentives or accountabilities, rather than interventions that rely on training and building individual capacity of informal providers. Yet the research in this area is not well

Table 9.2 Proportion of positive outcomes from studies involving informal private providers according to type of intervention strategy, among stronger study designs

Intervention strategy	Percentage positive
Training alone	21%
Training plus other interventions	58%
Training of trainers	71%
Supply provision	63%
Franchise	44%
Branding/social marketing	76%
Regulation	53%
Reinforcement with printed media	61%
Financial incentives, subsidies	55%
Supervision	59%
Referral system	71%

Source: Shah *et al.* (2010).
Note: Stronger study designs include randomized controlled trials, pre-post studies with controls, and case-control studies ($n = 26$).

Table 9.3 Proportion of positive outcomes from studies involving informal private providers according to the number of interventions

Number of intervention strategies	Percentage positive
One	48%
Two	50%
Three	65%
Four	88%
Total	56%

Source: Shah *et al.* (2010).

developed, and further understanding of the effects of such strategies will require more rigorous research designs.

The need for much better information on the functioning of health markets

Systematic evidence about what works and what fails, and why, is sparse. Several reasons are reported and include weak stewardship of the private sector, non-evaluation of programs and non-publication of results (Hanson *et al.*, 2008). Researchers have called for high-quality and systematic experimental and quasi-experimental evaluations[20] of private-sector innovations that would focus on both outcomes and processes (Hanson *et al.*, 2008; Koehlmoos *et al.*, 2009). Primary outcomes to be measured include access, quality of care, health outcomes, adverse effects and degree of financial and corporate sustainability. Contextual factors need to be taken into account. Those include socio-economic, demographic and environmental factors as well as the structure of the health market where the innovation takes place (e.g. healthcare delivery structure, health workforce, drugs and equipment supplies, law and regulations, competitive environment). The quality of a piece of research is usually assessed by the level of control the researcher has on implementation, contextual factors and key actors involved.

While we certainly recognize the great value of such studies and also advocate for them when feasible, we suggest that other types of research methodology such as rigorous case studies and action research can also significantly contribute to the learning process that needs to happen with market-based innovations and international initiatives in the private health sector. Health services innovations, however, involve many parallel changes, multiple actors and stakeholders, and are often very contextual. They grow and expand with or without the support of the public health authorities or the international donor community in mostly unregulated environments. Because of this diversity, complexity and context specificity, the research question is less about what works and more about how and why it works (or does not), and what can be done to foster an environment that helps the expansion of market-based innovations while minimizing unintended impact or side effects. The methodological question here is whether the research and evaluation design allows for understanding how these factors influence the results and highlight intermediate factors (rather than whether research is in full control of those factors). An innovation can rarely be seen as an autonomous unit. Rather, it involves a system of actions and a net of actors from policymakers, suppliers and competitors to patients that interact among themselves and whose situations change simultaneously in related and unrelated ways. Such research also needs to adopt a multi-perspective approach: it aims at developing knowledge and skills to better understand, monitor, improve and replicate innovations while reducing potential unintended effects. It focuses on the how and the why of success and failure. It promotes sharing of lessons learned among entrepreneurs. Research also supports the view that public health authorities and governments should play a regulating and monitoring role to foster an environment in support for 'good' innovations. Other research stakeholders include the donor community, the pharmaceutical industry, clinicians, professional associations and many others. Research can also adopt a macroeconomic perspective and document the impact of innovations on the health markets (e.g. competition, prices, products and organizations' behavior).

Case studies, action research and mixed methods are increasingly considered as rigorous alternative research methods where the researchers cannot control implementation and contextual factors cannot be used. Those methods have the advantage of taking into account the context and the complexity of actors and interested groups involved in the innovations as well as parallel changes that usually happen at the same time and in diverse domains and levels. Feagin *et al.* (1991) said that case studies 'strive towards a holistic understanding of cultural systems of action', a phrase also applicable to action research. The unit of analysis is a system of actions, rather than individuals. Case studies and action research enable the adoption of a multi-perspective approach. They use retrospective and/or prospective qualitative and quantitative methods. They enable the researcher to enter the world of the entrepreneurs and get an insider's information about the 'how' and the 'why', and contribute to the general body of knowledge. Action research goes further and uniquely empowers entrepreneurs and researchers to improve business models and adjust for unintended effects. They learn by doing. Entrepreneurs benefit from advice from external consultants who have accumulated relevant knowledge and experience from working on other innovations. Action research addresses the 'theory–practice' gap and acts as a self-regulating mechanism and motivates entrepreneurs to address unintended effects. 'The strength of action research is its ability to influence practice positively while simultaneously gathering data to share with a wider audience' (Meyer, 2000). To ensure the validity of findings, those methods can use various strategies, including triangulation with data, investigators, theories and methodologies (Feagin *et al.*, 1991). Findings based on a number of cases demonstrate the potential for replication and for drawing general conclusions (Noor, 2008).

The main challenge of those two research methods, and inherent to the way innovations develop, is access to information. This can be challenging for market-based innovations that operate in a competitive environment. Additionally, action research will only work if entrepreneurs 'perceive the need for change and are willing to play an active part in the process and the change process' (Meyer, 2000). Donors should make it a priority to include rigorous research in every grant so that research becomes part of routine practice. Public health authorities, donors and researchers, while building knowledge and skills, will be in a better position to effectively interact with the private sector and become more relevant and enabling partners.

Notes

1 The Center for Health Market Innovations (CHMI) initiative, funded by the Rockefeller Foundation and the Bill and Melinda Gates Foundation, has been building a database of innovative health initiatives since 2010 (http://healthmarketinnovations.org). The Nextbillion.net platform (www.nextbillion.net) brings together social entrepreneurs, business leaders, NGOs, policymakers and academics to exchange information about innovative business models. It has published a number of case studies in health. Dominic Montagu, of the Global Health Group at the University of California, San Francisco, has developed a list of private-sector initiatives (www.ps4h.org/resources). The IFC, in collaboration with the Gates Foundation, commissioned an overview of health care markets in Africa (IFC, 2007). Ashoka is one of the leading networks of social entrepreneurs. USAID has leading networks of social entrepreneurs. Finally, USAID has funded PSP-One and then SHOPS, programs for private-sector development in health that focus on reproductive health services (www.psp-one.com).
2 For example, Business for Health in Ghana, Living Goods in Uganda, Janani in India, or BRAC in Bangladesh.
3 For example, Aravind and Narayana Hrudayala in India.
4 For example, ProSalud provides primary, secondary and tertiary services to its patients, ranging from community outreach activities to services provided through its referral

hospitals. The CFWshops franchise started its operations with two levels of care: outlets run by a trained community health worker, and small clinics run by a nurse. Referral mechanisms have been put in place from the outlets to the clinics.

5 For example, Bio24 in Senegal and the Radmed Diagnostic Centre in Nigeria.

6 This is the case, for example, for Business for Health, Living Goods or CareShops. ProSalud has a cost recovery of 98 per cent (discussion with Carlos Cuellar, Abt Associates).

7 For example, Farmacias Similares pharmacies and ProSalud are located in poor neighborhoods in urban and peri-urban areas.

8 Business for Health in Ghana, Living Goods in Uganda, and the Shatki entrepreneurs in India.

9 The CFWshops franchise was started by the Health Store Foundation, funded by a US lawyer.

10 In India, Hindustan Liver Ltd partnered with self-help groups to start a network of women entrepreneurs to distribute its products in rural areas. Farmacias Similares was set up by a generic drug manufacturer to expand sales coverage to low-income areas through quality services. The network now comprises 3,000 pharmacies throughout Mexico.

11 This has led the Ghana Social Marketing Foundation, after years of successful family planning and social marketing activities, to create the CareShop franchise, a network of 270 licensed chemical sellers. Population Services International (PSI) and Marie Stopes International started several franchise initiatives for the same reasons (e.g. PSI Top Réseau Network and PSI Sun Quality Health).

12 K-MET started as an association of for-profit medical practitioners from peri-urban and rural areas in Kenya.

13 An example of accreditation scheme is the ADDOShops initiative in Tanzania. Accreditation to the ADDOs network is granted to those who meet and keep predefined standards of quality.

14 For example, Greenstar and Blue Star.

15 For example, CFWshops and CareShops.

16 The success factors of ProSalud and Aravind, for example, lie in their high-quality delivery system, including standardization and strict quality control.

17 For example, Aravind organizes community outreach activities to increase awareness about its services and build trust. PSI initiates media campaigns to promote its franchise brands. Farmacias Similares has built a strong image of quality around the person of Dr Simi and his motto 'Lo mismo pero más barato' (the same but cheaper).

18 For example, ProSalud places patients at the centre of its services, training and organization. Services are provided in the evening and over the weekend. LifeSpring in India emphasizes the importance of treatment of each patient's tailored needs. Patients are called 'clients', as in a hotel.

19 ProSalud has priority targets to reduce patients' waiting time; Aravind provides free transportation to go to hospital to referred patients; Business for Health (set up by Freedom from Hunger in Ghana) and Living Goods (Uganda) bring products and services to families directly in their home.

20 For example, randomized or non-randomized controlled trials, interrupted time series, controlled before and after series.

References

Agha, S., Karim, A. M., Balal, A. and Sosler, S. (2007) 'The impact of a reproductive health franchise on client satisfaction in rural Nepal', *Health Policy and Planning*, 22 (5): 320–328

Cuellar, C. J., Newbrander, W. C. and Price, G. (2000) *Extending Access to Health Care through Public/Private Partnerships: The PROSALUD Experience*, MSH Publications, Cambridge, MA

Feagin, J., Orum, A. and Sjoberg, G. (1991) *A Case for Case Study*, University of North Carolina Press, Chapel Hill

Hanson, K., Gilson, L., Goodman, C., Mills, A., Smith, R., Feachem, R., Feachem, N. S., Koehlmoos, T. P. and Kinlaw, H. (2008) 'Is private health care the answer to the health problems of the world's poor?', *PLoS Medicine*, 5 (11): 1528–1532

Hennink, M. and Clements, S. (2004) 'Impact of franchised family planning clinics in urban poor areas in Pakistan', Applications and Policy Working Paper A04/16, Southampton Statistical Sciences Research Institute, University of Southampton. Online, available at: http://eprints.soton.ac.uk/12491/1/12491-01.pdf (accessed 19 April 2012)

HLSP Institute (2004) 'Private sector participation in health'. Online, available at: www.hlspinstitute.org/projects/?mode=type&id=15043 (accessed 2 July 2008)

International Finance Corporation (IFC) (2007) *The Business of Health in Africa*, World Bank Group, IFC Health and Education Department, Washington, DC. Online, available at: www.ifc.org/ifcext/healthinafrica.nsf/Content/FullReport

Koehlmoos, T. P., Gazi, R., Hossain, S. S. and Zaman, K. (2009) 'The effect of social franchising on access to and quality of health services in low- and middle-income countries', *Cochrane Database of Systematic Reviews*, Issue I. Art. No.: CD007136

Leonard, K. (2002) 'When both states and markets fail: asymmetric information and the role of NGOs in African health care', *International Review of Law and Economics*, 22 (1): 61–80

Meyer, J. (2000) 'Using qualitative methods in health related action research', *British Medical Journal*, 320: 178–181

Mills, A., Brugha, R., Hanson, K. and McPake, B. (2002) 'What can be done about the private health sector in low-income countries?', *Bulletin of the World Health Organization*, 80 (4): 325–330.

Montagu, D., Prata, N., Campbell, M. M., Walsh, J. and Orero, S. (2005) *Kenya: Reaching the Poor Through the Private Sector: A Network Model for Expanding Access to Reproductive Health Services*, HNP (The World Bank). Online, available at: http://site resources.worldbank.org/HEALTHNUTRITIONANDPOPULATION/Resources/281 627-1095698140167/KenyaMontaguFinal.pdf (accessed 2 July 2008)

Noor, K. B. M. (2008) 'Case study: a strategic research methodology', *American Journal of Applied Science*, 5 (11): 1602–1604

Patouillard, E., Goodman, C. A., Hanson, K. G. and Mills, A. J. (2007) 'Can working with the private for-profit sector improve utilization of quality health services by the poor? A systematic review of the literature', *International Journal for Equity in Health*, 6: 17

Peters, D. H., Mirchandani, G. G. and Hansen, P. M. (2004) 'Strategies for engaging the private sector in sexual and reproductive health: how effective are they?', *Health Policy and Planning*, 19 (suppl. 1): i5–i21

Plautz, A., Meekers, D. and Neukom, J. (2003) 'The impact of the Madagascar TOP Réseau: social marketing program on sexual behavior and use of reproductive health services', PSI Working Paper 57, Population Services International, Washington, DC

Population Services International (PSI) (2007) *Cambodia: Family Planning TRaC-M Study Evaluating Quality of Care Among Social Franchising Providers in Kampong Thom and Kampot*, The PSI Dashboard, March. Online, available at: http://www.psi.org/ sites/default/files/publication_files/724-cambodia_trac-m_fp_smrs.pdf (accessed 19 April 2012)

Prata, N., Montagu, D. and Jefferys, E. (2005) 'Private sector, human resources and health franchising in Africa', *Bulletin of the World Health Organization*, 83: 274–279

PSP-One (2006) 'Private provider networks: the role of viability in expanding the supply of reproductive health and family planning services'. Online, available at: www.abt associates.com/reports/private_provider_networks_0406.pdf (accessed 19 April 2012)

Reinikka, R. and Svensson, J. (2003) 'Working for God? Evaluating service delivery of religious not-for-profit health care providers in Uganda' World Bank Policy Research Working Paper 3058, World Bank, Washington, DC. Online, available at: http://papers.ssrn.com/sol3/papers.cfm?abstract_id=636420 (accessed 3 July 2008)

Rolfe, B., Leshabari, S., Rutta, F. and Murray, S. F. (2008) 'The crisis in human resources for health care and the potential of a "retired" workforce: case study of the independent midwifery sector in Tanzania', *Health Policy and Planning*, 23 (2): 137–149

Shah, N. M., Brieger, W. and Peters, D. H. (2010) 'Can interventions improve health services from informal private providers in low and middle-income countries? A comprehensive review of the literature', *Health Policy and Planning*, 10: 1–13. doi:10.1093/heapol/czq074

Shawn, C. (2001) 'External assessment of health care', *British Medical Journal*, 322: 851–854

Sigonda-Ndomondo, M., Kowero, O., Alphonce, E., Mbwasi, R., Shirima, R., Frankiewicz, C., Taylor, M., Heltzer, N. and Clark, M. (2003) *Accredited Drug Dispensing Outlets: A Novel Public–Private Partnership*, Management Sciences for Health, Tanzania

Stephenson, R., Tsui, A. O., Sulzbach, S., Bardsley, P., Bekele, G., Giday, T., Ahmed, R., Gopalkrishnan, G. and Feyesitan, B. (2004) 'Franchising reproductive health services', *Health Services Research*, 39: 2053–2080

Tibandebage, P. and Mackintosh, M. (2005) 'The market shaping of charges, trust and abuse: health care transactions in Tanzania', *Social Science and Medicine*, 61: 1385–1396

WHO (2007) 'Public policy and franchising reproductive health: current evidence and future directions', Guidance from a technical consultation meeting, WHO, USAID, and PSP-One. Online, available at: www.who.int/reproductivehealth/publications/health_systems/9789241596021/en/index.html (accessed 19 April 2012)

10 A review of ICT innovations by private-sector providers in developing countries

Henry Lucas

There has been much discussion of the role that recent advances in information and communications technology (ICT) can play in improving health provider performance, though as yet there seems to be little reliable, independently verified evidence to support the optimism of those who initially viewed these technologies as offering 'a revolution in global healthcare management' (Séror, 2001, p. 1). A number of literature reviews have noted the paucity of rigorous evaluations, especially in developing countries (Blaya *et al.*, 2010; Kahn *et al.*, 2010), and one recent study suggests that research reports often paint a picture of 'unexpected and limited outcomes, failed and abandoned projects' (Halford *et al.*, 2010).

In particular, limited systematic attention has been given to the application of ICT by private (whether for-profit or not-for-profit) providers in developing countries, with most of the international agencies concerned with these issues tending to focus on public-sector innovations (e.g. Chetley, 2006; WHO, 2006). A recent report commissioned by UNICEF on the use of mobile phones in development interventions targeting the poor highlights that, in spite of frequent claims to the contrary, there has in fact been limited private-sector engagement. The report argues that when major companies are involved in such interventions, the engagement is typically with small corporate social responsibility departments which have 'small budgets and limited decision-making power' (Boakye *et al.*, 2010, p. 2). It suggests that many operators are willing to collaborate only if there is a clear potential for the development, possibly over an extended period, of a service that will provide a return on investment comparable to that available elsewhere.

It has long been argued that the successful implementation of innovations in the private sector typically requires a receptive 'technological system' (Stewart, 1977), where required inputs are readily available and delivered outputs satisfy existing demands. One reason that some developments in ICT have had such a major impact is that they addressed long-felt and well-understood *needs*. Small businesses, including those in the health sector, have always recognized the value of being able to communicate reliably and in a timely fashion with both suppliers and customers. The arrival of the mobile phone addressed this specific requirement to an extent previously unimaginable, allowing instant communication even in some of the most remote and least developed areas. Similarly, it has been long understood that maintaining current, reliable and easily accessible data on stocks, customers, activities and finance could be enormously valuable in making good management decisions. Again, the development of relatively inexpensive personal computers and user-friendly software has made it possible for such activities to be undertaken much more efficiently and reliably.

As in the design of health services, it is important to distinguish *needs* from *wants* in the area of new technology. The diversity of proposed applications in the health sector is very impressive. Reviews of the recent literature (e.g. WHO, 2010) indicate enthusiasm for the value of ICT in areas that include:

- patient registrations and appointments or admissions;
- health management information 'systems' (integrated to a greater or lesser extent) covering population health status, health services, human resources, finance, infrastructure, pharmaceuticals, clinical laboratory and testing services, etc.;
- patient-focused electronic health/medical records (HER/EMR);
- clinical decision-making support software;
- online clinical and pharmaceutical reference manuals;
- provider-initiated patient information and appointment or treatment reminders;
- disease-specific networks of patients, carers, advocates and providers;
- remote diagnosis and consultation;
- remote population and health service data collection;
- health promotion;
- health advisory services.

Many of these applications have seen a plethora of government- or donor-funded 'pilot exercises'. However, very few survive when funding is withdrawn. On the other hand, many low-key, relatively uncomplicated applications have spread rapidly within the private health sector, as elsewhere, mostly going unreported and unremarked (Kaplan, 2006). They tend to emerge into public awareness only if they are taken up by the specialist media, donor agencies or curious academics. Three illustrative examples originate from South Africa. On Cue, a company established by a TB specialist, uses a simple computerized telephone system to send text messages reminding patients to take medication at predetermined times.[1] SIMpill[2] takes this approach one stage further by manufacturing a drug dispenser that automatically monitors and records patient self-medication and sends an SMS message to a carer if there is serious non-compliance. Cell-Life[3] (Skinner *et al.*, 2007; Khan, 2004), a not-for-profit organization supported by Vodacom, provided mobile phones to a team of locally recruited counsellors who monitor the treatment and health status of around 800 HIV/AIDS patients. Healthcare staff at a collaborating clinic can access this information via a central database and intervene if problems arise. A similar intervention has been running for some time in India, where paramedics and community volunteers attached to the Bombay Leprosy Project have been provided with mobile phones and pagers to link patients with clinic doctors, for example to reach rapid decisions on the need for emergency treatment.[4]

On a larger scale, the Health Information and Service call centre, available to GrameenPhone mobile phone subscribers in Bangladesh (GrameenPhone, 2006), is said to be widely used not only by those with health problems but also by informal health providers when they have doubts about a diagnosis or treatment. The service is reported to be responding to some 10,000 callers each day (Mechael, 2009). The Grameen Foundation in Ghana is also collaborating with the Columbia University School of Public Health to explore a role for low-cost mobile phones to provide health information to rural communities, with an initial focus on maternal and newborn health. The 'Mobile Technologies for Community Health' project,[5] funded by the Gates Foundation, will similarly attempt to support community health workers providing antenatal and neonatal care through mobile phone-based links to the district level (Mechael, 2009).

Voxiva, a communications company that has pioneered the use of information systems based around mobile phones, has played the central role, with national and international donor funding, in establishing a number of regional health networks. The Health Watch disease surveillance project in Tamil Nadu[6] was set up following the tsunami disaster in 2004 and a system whereby rural healthcare providers use mobile phones to provide routine assessment data on high-risk pregnancies to centrally based senior staff is operating in the Ucayali region of Peru.[7] The mobile phone giant Nokia has recently entered into a partnership with the Brazilian government to provide a similar mobile phone-based network for community health workers providing services to the indigenous population. Funded by the UN Foundation and the Clinton Global Initiative, the MobiSUS project[8] aims to provide a system for collecting and disseminating health information from some of the most remote areas.

Interestingly, a similar intervention, named 'TeleDoc', was piloted in India as early as 2001 by the private Ayurvedic treatment provider Jiva (Singh, 2006). Initially supported by a grant from the Soros Foundation, this project provided rural healthcare workers with mobile phones or personal data assistants (PDAs) programmed to record and transmit diagnostic data. A panel of doctors in Delhi then analysed these data to determine appropriate treatment. Prescribed medicines were delivered to the patient's home by project field workers. This project appears to have been suspended when grant funding ceased.

SMS applications

One rapidly expanding area of activity, probably driven by the relatively low cost, is the use of text messaging for health applications (e.g. United Nations, 2011). It is possible to establish for-profit business models in this area, as demonstrated by mDhil,[9] an apparently successful enterprise that uses SMS to provide health information about common health conditions to some 150,000 subscribers in India. However, most examples appear to involve collaborations between not-for-profit organizations or social enterprises and private mobile phone companies. For example, in the Mbarara district of Uganda the AIDS Information Centre and a local mobile phone provider, Zain, are working with the NGO 'Text to Change' to provide short health promotion messages relating to HIV/AIDS (IRIN PlusNews, 2008).

Towards the end of 2008 the not-for-profit Poptech network, which includes many leading ICT entrepreneurs and technologists, launched Project Masiluleke, employing mobile technology to encourage HIV testing and antiretroviral (ARV) treatment in South Africa.[10] This project is part of the Poptech Accelerator programme, which aims to support major technical innovations by providing an appropriate combination of project management, finance, media coverage and corporate partnerships. In the initial stages, around 1 million local-language text messages each day are being broadcast over the mobile phone network. These encourage individuals who feel they may be at risk to call government-funded HIV call centres. These provide advice and, where necessary, referral to regional healthcare centres capable of providing voluntary HIV testing and counselling, TB screening, and treatment with ARVs and TB medication.

One novel aspect of the latter project is that it makes use of 'Please Call Me' text messaging, a free SMS service widely available in South Africa and elsewhere in the continent. This substantially reduces the overall cost. A controversial second phase of the project will make available low-cost HIV self-testing kits designed to be used in conjunction with a mobile phone-based counselling service. Poptech argues that the known risks of self-testing are outweighed by the scale of the problem in South Africa and report that the approach has been welcomed by health authorities. The final component will use TxtAlert,[11] an open-source[12] mobile phone application, to send routine SMS reminders of clinic appointments to those receiving treatment for HIV/AIDS and/or TB.

In Mexico a communications billionaire, Carlos Slim Helú, has launched the VidaNET system[13] (Feder, 2010), which provides an automated compliance service via mobile phone for HIV-positive individuals. After registering with the system and providing details of their treatment schedule, they receive a short text message whenever medication is due. The service is funded jointly by the not-for-profit Carso Health Institute and Telcel, which is owned by Latin America's largest mobile phone company, América Móvil, in which Mr Helú is a major shareholder. The aim is to extend the service to those suffering from diabetes and heart disease. In a recent donor-funded initiative, Cell-Life has focused on reducing mother-to-child transmission of HIV in South Africa.[14] SMS is used to encourage compliance with prevention programmes by sending text messages over a ten-week period to remind HIV-positive mothers about appointments and medication. The cost per mother is around $1.50. Unlike many other such initiatives, a serious evaluation is currently being undertaken. A randomized controlled trial has thus far indicated that mothers in the programme are more likely to bring their babies for HIV testing (United Nations, 2011).

Kiwanja.net[15] is a not-for-profit organization that aims to facilitate innovative applications of mobile technology by NGOs. It has developed an open-source[16] software product (FrontlineSMS) that allows a cluster of even the most basic (cheapest) mobile phones to be linked via a standard laptop computer without an internet connection, such that messages can be sent either to individuals or to groups of individuals. There have been numerous applications in areas including training, mobile payment systems and legal services. A recent development, which does require somewhat more advanced[17] (and expensive) mobile phones, allows downloading of simple questionnaire forms that can be completed and transmitted as SMS text. There is a particular focus on healthcare applications (FrontlineSMS: Medic) including electronic medical records (PatientView). It is intended to extend the system to include remote diagnostics and mapping of services. The software is provided free of charge to non-profit organizations.

An ongoing debate familiar from other contexts concerns the relative advantages of making best use of established technologies or seeking to plan for the advances that are expected to be available in the 'near' future. The debate is often constructed as a choice between investing in innovations, such as those described above, that extend and improve the use of voice and text messaging based on existing second-generation (2G), relatively low-cost[18] GSM[19] mobile phone networks, or developing new, potentially far more sophisticated, applications ('apps') that rely on the third-generation (3G) high-speed data networks required to access the internet (Selanikio, 2010). In practice, the options are far more nuanced. The move from 2G to 3G networks had at least two intermediary steps that had the potential to deliver higher speeds and enhanced services.[20] A further complication is the development of an enormous variety of mobile phones that cannot access the internet but can be connected to laptop computers for data transfer and are able to run a range of useful software applications (for example using the keypad for completion of a stored survey questionnaire).[21] They are typically priced somewhere between basic mobiles and smartphones.

One argument often used in favour of the 'current technology' approach is the enormous existing investment in 2G mobiles, even in some of the poorest countries. For example, the penetration ratio (number of subscriptions per 100 inhabitants) is over 40 in Nigeria and over 30 in Tanzania and Zambia. Coverage of GSM networks is over 50 per cent for Africa as a whole and over 40 per cent even in rural areas. With the notable exception of South Africa, internet access in many African countries is limited to less (and in some case considerably less) than 5 per cent of the population (UNCTAD, 2009). Moreover, the communications infrastructure investment required to radically change this situation is almost certainly not affordable by many governments and not commercially attractive to private companies.

On the other hand, more expensive mobile phones do allow applications that go beyond those allowed by traditional voice and text messaging capabilities. The not-for-profit company Datadyne[22] has attracted considerable attention worldwide (and funding from the United Nations Foundation, Vodafone Foundation, and World Bank) by developing a mobile phone-based data collection system, EpiSurveyor (Schuster and Perez Brito, 2011). Survey forms are designed on a desktop or laptop computer and then transferred to a Java-enabled mobile phone for use in the field. Data can then be transferred from the phone to a remote web server or local computer for analysis. The software has been targeted at the health sector and undergone successful reasonably large-scale pilot exercises in Malawi and Kenya. One interesting aspect of this innovation is that while most users can download and run the software at no cost, a substantial subscription fee ($5,000 per year) is required to remove limits on sample sizes and number of questions per form, and to gain access to technical support services. Datadyne argues that requesting fees from a minority of users is necessary for a sustainable business model, allowing it to subsidize smaller-scale users.

The potential of smartphones

The current generation of mobile smartphones[23] are essentially hand-held computers, which implies that many apparently innovative developments simply involve the adaptation of existing software applications. Many companies sell apps that allow the use of mobiles to measure or monitor heart rate, respiratory rate, blood pressure and body temperature, issue automatic reminders on medication schedules and provide access to internet-based medical advice and reference materials.[24] Detailed eye examinations can be undertaken in remote locations using a mobile phone attachment developed by the Massachusetts Institute of Technology.[25] The US company Qualcomm[26] is one among a number of companies that have developed technology for automatic monitoring of blood glucose levels using two very small metal strips that are inserted under the skin and transmit blood glucose information to the patient's mobile phone, alerting both the patient and their doctor to any development that requires attention.

Such developments have contributed to major advances in the area of tele-medicine: remote diagnosis and consultation (Hersh *et al.*, 2006). Afridoctor[27] is an application designed for upmarket Nokia smartphones. It was developed by Blueworld Communities, a South African media company concerned with the development of social networking web technologies. The novel service offered is that customers can send a photograph of a skin condition, bite or injury and receive professional advice on treatment from a panel of doctors. The application can also be used to locate providers, using Google Maps, transmit a distress message with location information to a specified relative, check common symptoms to assess the need to see a provider, and obtain basic first aid guidance. While the application has won awards from Nokia, it has apparently been little used within Africa, given that few people have the required third-generation mobiles.[28] Another smartphone application for personal diabetes management has been developed by Entra Health Systems, a company specializing in healthcare management technology. This involves a wireless link between a blood glucose meter and a smartphone.[29] Both patients and providers can access time series data on test results to assess the need for behaviour or treatment modification.

A key constraint on improvement of rural health services in many countries has been the inability of providers to undertake the laboratory tests required for reliable diagnosis of even very common diseases. For example, there is considerable evidence as to the over-diagnosis of malaria in many countries (Amexo *et al.*, 2004). In many cases, microscopic examination of blood or tissue samples could greatly improve diagnosis of many haematological and infectious diseases, but few facilities can afford the initial cost, have the required diagnostic skills or can provide the necessary environment for the effective use and maintenance of a traditional microscopy service. At least two recent innovations have addressed this concern. The CellScope[30] project (Breslauer *et al.*, 2009) has been implemented by staff of the Blum Centre at Berkeley, a foundation established with funding from the investment banker Richard Blum. It involves the use of a relatively standard light microscope mounted on a mobile camera phone. This device can generate both normal bright-field and fluorescence photomicrographs using the normal detector in the phone. These can then be transmitted to a remote laboratory where both visual diagnosis and automated image analysis – for example, the counting of bacilli – can be undertaken. A very different approach has been taken by the Ozcan Research Group,[31] part of the California NanoSystems Institute at the University of California, Los Angeles (UCLA). This uses a small holographic microscope that has no lenses, lasers or other sensitive optical components. It is attached directly to the camera unit of the mobile, with illumination from a light-emitting diode being reflected from each object to create a holographic signature on the standard detector. As above, the resulting signals are transmitted to a diagnostic centre where the images are reconstructed from these signatures (Tseng *et al.*, 2010).

ICT and health management

An innovative mobile phone-based exercise was undertaken in Tanzania by IBM, Vodafone and Novatis working in collaboration with the Ministry of Health and Social Welfare and the Roll Back Malaria partnership[32] (Barrington *et al.*, 2010). Providers in 129 facilities, whose location was identified using Google Maps, submitted weekly toll-free text messages over mobile phones supplied by Vodafone, detailing their current stock of malaria drugs. This information was relayed to a central database in the United Kingdom, where IBM software (LotusLive) generated routine reports, identified potential stock-outs and issued delivery instructions for deliveries by Novartis. This replaced the existing inventory tracking system, which had resulted in 40 per cent of clinics being out of medicines at any given time.

Sproxil[33] describes itself as a 'privately backed' social enterprise. It originated in Nigeria with support from Intel Capital[34] and provides a mobile phone-based 'track and trace' system that allows wholesalers, retailers and consumers to check the authenticity of medicines. The system uses the asymmetric or 'public key' encryption approach commonly adopted for internet transactions. Labels containing a 'scratch code' similar to those used to purchase pay-as-you-go mobile phone time can be applied to packaging at different levels down to the individual tablet strip. A telephone call to a central server allows authentication of the code and tracking of the product through the supply chain where required, for example if a product recall is necessary. For manufacturers and distributors the system provides a potentially valuable marketing information database. The labels can also be used for advertising and product promotion exercises. A related innovation is led by the mPedigree Network,[35] a not-for-profit enterprise based in Ghana that is attempting to build an international consortium of pharmaceutical and ICT companies to develop an industry-wide mobile authentication service. Pilot exercises have taken place in Nigeria, Ghana[36] and Kenya.[37]

Reliable information on the use of computer-based management systems by health providers in developing countries is even scarcer than that on mobile phone applications. However, the importance of a receptive environment is well illustrated by recent reviews of two broadly comparable innovatory exercises in Ghana and Mexico by the World Resources Institute (WRI). The retail pharmacy chain Careshop was established by a for-profit subsidiary of the Ghana Social Marketing Foundation (GSMF) in 2002 (Segrè and Tran, 2008). It is a franchise of licensed retailers of over-the-counter drugs, operating under GSMF guidelines that are intended to improve the quality, accessibility and affordability of essential medicines. When a donation of 100 new computers was received, they were allocated over time to franchisees on the basis of their performance. However, the great majority were never used, and at the time of the WRI review they were typically either not in working order or not connected to an electricity supply. Their owners were theoretically interested in using the computers to record sales data but had been deterred by practical difficulties or cost implications. They apparently valued the computers highly but only as symbols that they could put on display to indicate the success of their business.

On the other hand, the Mexican pharmacy franchise Mi Farmacita Nacional was said to have fully integrated computerized patient records and inventory control into its management processes (Coronado et al., 2007). Though Mi Farmacita is a fully for-profit company, it has adopted a social entrepreneurship model similar to that of Careshop, aiming to provide essential drugs and health services to low-income populations. Each franchisee is responsible for hiring a relatively inexperienced, though qualified, doctor. Each time these doctors diagnose and write a prescription, details are entered onto a centralized computer system via a terminal located in the facility, generating the data required for monitoring professional performance. The computer is also used for inventory management, allowing franchisees to monitor their stocks and place orders. The associated sales database can be accessed across the franchise chain, and franchisees are encouraged to compare product sales and prices to promote competition.

First Care[38] is a healthcare initiative by Rural Technology and Business Incubator (RTBI), a society set up by the Indian Institute of Technology to promote technology-based business ventures in rural areas. It aims to create a network of trained and accredited primary care providers by working with rural medical practitioners, informal private providers who typically operate as solo practices in rural communities. They form the largest cadre of private health providers in rural India and are by far the most popular source of care for the rural poor. First Care regards ICT as absolutely central to its project. It plans to link clinics with internet- and mobile phone-enabled kiosks that will provide access both to distance learning materials and to physicians and hospitals that are willing to offer advice, laboratory testing and referral support. It also intends to introduce personal computer and mobile phone-based record-keeping systems that will allow quantity and quality monitoring of services. At present, just one pilot activity is under way with a small group of rural medical practitioners in a rural area of Tamil Nadu.

An alternative approach to rural health care in India, deliberately bypassing informal providers, is being piloted by Drishtee,[39] a for-profit franchise organization that aims to use ICT to promote entrepreneurship in rural areas. It has established a network of around 1,000 kiosks across six states, with each kiosk having a catchment population of around 1,200 households. It was initially focused on providing access to a range of key information sources – for example, government records and commodity prices – and assisting applications for licences, certificates and benefits. Drishtee has also set up a range of training courses, particularly in computer literacy and spoken English. In 2006, working with Microsoft India (Drishtee Foundation, 2010), it set up kiosk cooperatives in a small number of villages in the Madhubani district, one of the poorest in Bihar State, to provide videoconferencing facilities that allow diagnosis and prescription by doctors in an NGO health centre in the capital, Patna. This involves the use of a recently developed remote diagnostics unit that captures blood pressure, heart and lung sounds, oxygen saturation, temperature and pulse rate. The health centre maintains computerized patient records for those using the kiosk and has links to a referral hospital that can undertake laboratory tests and provide a referral service. The kiosks can also be used to arrange purchase of prescribed drugs from an accredited pharmacy.

A third variant on this theme is currently being piloted in Pakistan. Sehat First, a joint venture between d.o.t.z. Technologies (a social enterprise) and the Acumen Fund (a non-profit venture capital fund), has set up ICT-based health centres in five locations in Bin Qasim Town in the south-eastern part of Karachi. These first started to receive patients in April 2008, and the ambition is to establish 500 centres across Pakistan by 2012.[40] Again, the model is based on franchised health centres, which in this case incorporate a multipurpose telecentre, pharmacy and general store, with the aim of ensuring financial viability. They are targeted at areas with very limited formal health services and aim to provide basic care, pharmaceuticals and a tele-consultancy service similar to that envisaged by Drishtee. Support for these services is provided by partnership agreements with Aga Khan Medical Services and Unilever Pakistan.

As the above examples show, the general franchise model can take a variety of forms. One key dimension of this flexibility is the degree to which they are centrally directed and regulated. ICTs have greatly extended the possibilities for both centralization and decentralization. The availability of reliable communications and a stand-alone computer in each facility has the potential to increase the ability of local managers to be self-reliant, for example maintaining their own supplier, customer and inventory databases, and keeping track of their own sales and finances. On the other hand, the same equipment can allow a central authority to undertake detailed monitoring of their activities.

An extreme example of the latter, though in a retail chain rather than a franchise operation, is provided by an independent evaluation study covering the period

1998–1999 of what was then the largest and most widely dispersed chain of private urban clinics in South Africa (Palmer *et al*., 2003). The clinics offered ambulatory care to patients, who either paid a flat fee or were members of an affiliated insurance scheme. The aim was to provide an attractive and trustworthy service, including on-site availability of doctors, laboratory tests, X-ray and ultrasound equipment, and drugs, at a price that would allow access to a wide range of urban workers, not only those in well-paid employment. The average cost per visit was around 42 rand (US$7). It would appear that the ICT system was a key factor in holding down costs and hence allowing the company to adopt this pricing policy. Each clinic was linked to the head office of the company over a computer network that handled both clinical and management information. On entry, a patient would initially be seen by a healthcare worker, who would enter personal details and symptoms into the computer network. This could access a database of more than 2,000 algorithms for diagnosis and treatment derived from the Cochrane Collaboration Reviews. The reliability of this database was central to the overall operation, given that computer-based diagnosis is not a trivial undertaking (Peters *et al*., 2006). Three outcomes were then possible. The health worker might use the information system to arrive at a diagnosis and recommended treatment; pass the patient on to a clinic nurse; or tell the patient that clinic was not able to assist them. A similar procedure would take place for patients referred to the nurse, except that in these cases an onward referral would be to a clinic doctor.

Healthcare workers, nurses and doctors were all expected to follow recommended treatment protocols, and decisions to act otherwise would be systematically recorded and reviewed by clinic and central managers. Any drugs provided from the clinic dispensary would be similarly compared to those implied by the recommended protocol and all deviations identified. The system thus allowed not only for routine clinical audits but detailed daily reports on revenues and costs relating to each patient visit. Overall, controlling access to clinic doctors, use of expert systems and strict adherence to protocols enabled staff costs to be less than half, and drug costs around a quarter, of those at comparable private general practices. The independent evaluation reported favourably on both the cost and quality of services provided.

Some might argue that the clinic chain exhibited two common characteristics of private-sector engagement in service provision: 'cherry-picking' areas where treatment was relatively straightforward and profitable, leaving the public sector to deal with the rest (Pollack, 2001); and deskilling staff by requiring them to follow the dictates of expert systems (Hanlon *et al*., 2005). These complaints are familiar from discussions around European healthcare systems, as are the counter-arguments: private provision in selected areas can 'reduce the overall burden' on the public sector, allowing a focus on areas of greatest need; and services should be run in the best interests of patients, not providers. This is not the place to address these long-running debates. The key observation for the present discussion is the crucial enabling role played by the computer system in the implementation of the adopted business model and in the fine-tuning of that model in pursuit of profitability. The example suggests that ICT may sharpen the debate around public versus private provision by increasing the range of strategies open to private companies seeking to establish profitable investments in the health sector.

As indicated, the model described above is crucially dependent on the use of accurate diagnostic software. This has become a rapidly expanding area of specialization for software companies and there are a considerable number of competing products in this market. One of the more interesting, because the intention is to distribute copies free of charge in developing countries, is NxOpinion. This was developed by the non-profit Robertson Research Institute[41] in collaboration with Microsoft Research. It is a real-time diagnostic tool intended to assist the diagnosis of around 500 illnesses and forms part of an integrated software package that also supports electronic health records (EHRs) and performance monitoring. Thus far, it has been piloted by missionary hospitals in the Dominican Republic and by a medical NGO, Doctors on Call for Service,[42] in the Democratic Republic of Congo. In 2008 the Elaj Group, which provides medical services in Saudi Arabia, the United Arab Emirates, Qatar and Egypt, signed a memorandum of understanding to distribute and promote the software, initially within its own centres and then to providers in Libya, Tunisia and Morocco.

Finally, the 'telecentre' or 'tele-kiosk' concept provides an interesting example of the possibilities and potential pitfalls of collaborative partnerships that extended general mobile communication initiatives into the health sector. These are primarily small- to medium-scale, typically private-sector, franchise enterprises with donor, NGO or government subsidies that aim to act as community communications centres combining telecommunications, the internet, email, fax, photocopying, printing and sometimes local radio, as in the Kothmale and Nakaseke examples (Fillip and Foote, 2007). The idea has proved extremely popular with governments, international agencies,[43] social entrepreneurs[44] and some private companies. In India, one apparently successful health application involved a collaboration between n-Logue Communications and Aravind Eye Hospitals (AEH). This provided outreach eye services to rural India via n-Logue's franchised network of privately owned, wirelessly connected village internet kiosks (Paul, 2004). Singh (2006) suggests that the relative effectiveness of this collaboration was in large part due to the very specific goals, organizational capacity and prior experience of AEH in providing services to poor rural populations. More recently, Microsoft's Project Saksham has agreed to set up 5,000 rural kiosks in India, providing a range of services including healthcare information, and has suggested an eventual target of 200,000 using satellite-based broadband.[45]

Many of the supporting organizations have indicated that the provision of health-related services should be a key component. Run by managers dedicated to serving the community, and employing trustworthy and benevolent local institutions and individuals – such as hospitals, health NGOs and local doctors – to mediate information flows, they might seem to provide at least a plausible route to bridging the digital divide in the health sector. However, this attractive scenario makes two key assumptions: first, that questions relating to health issues have but a single correct response on which all reputable mediators can agree; and second, that mediators will be both incorruptible and beyond the influence of local economic, social and political pressures. In practice, hospital doctors, for example, might well use internet resources to disparage remedies advocated by respected traditional healers or insist that people should not purchase drugs in markets run by local community leaders. They might take these positions on the basis of considered clinical judgement, professional hubris or commercial interest.

How would such disputes between potential mediators on health issues be conducted and resolved? Probably on the basis of local popular opinion and/or the degree of influence that the various parties can bring to bear on the telecentre management. Where governments or other donors are providing support, they too will clearly be in a position of influence but will typically not wish to be seen as micro-managing an institution explicitly identified as a local resource. The more successful the telecentre, the more it tends to lead debates on health issues and the greater the level of trust conferred on it by local community members, the more incentive there will be for capture by one or other local elite groups. The key point is the familiar one that health knowledge has a high value, not only in commercial terms but also in terms of social, cultural, religious and political currency – and valuable assets attract the attention of those who see potential advantage in their ownership. If telecentres are to become a serious source of health information, their governance structures should merit at least as much consideration as their technical capacity.

ICT and the health knowledge economy

The discussion so far has focused on the deliberate use of ICT by healthcare providers to improve access, efficiency or quality of services. However, these technologies have also very much changed the overall information environment within which providers operate. Bloom *et al.* (2008) suggest that health care is now best regarded as part of an emerging 'health knowledge economy'. For present purposes this might be conceptualized in terms of a real or quasi market in which multiple providers compete (or sometimes collude) to gain clients. Each such provider will claim that it can provide access to a stock of 'health knowledge', often embedded in medicinal products or other commodities, that has the potential[46] to improve the health status of an individual or population. Many proponents of ICT tend to focus only on issues relating to the distribution of such knowledge. They see the underlying objective in terms of removing infrastructure barriers to allow easier access to these multiple providers, adopting (usually implicitly) the assumption that a 'freer market' will in the long run allow the aggregate choices of rational individuals to determine the most desirable.

How does this work in practice? One obvious threat is that, as in the markets for other commodities, it is often the case that 'the medium is the message'. ICT provides enormously enhanced opportunities for much more attractive 'packaging' of health knowledge, greatly exacerbating traditional health sector concerns relating to asymmetric information and externalities. 'Big Pharma' provides the iconic image of those who have rushed to exploit these opportunities but, as the above discussion indicates, there are a host of other international, national and local-level players with a variety of motives that need to be considered. Even interventions led by well-intentioned NGOs, academics, social entrepreneurs, etc. may raise serious and interesting questions.

For example, one of the most common interventions adopted by such inter-mediaries is that of promoting a mobile phone-based service to allow access by poor rural households to a panel of qualified medical practitioners. The 'health knowledge' on offer via such mechanisms would typically be described as 'evidence based' and 'best practice'. However, even if we assume that all those involved are doing their best to provide 'good' information and advice, the fact that they may have very little knowledge of the specific local context in which that advice is to be implemented gives rise to a number of concerns. For example, physicians are trained to be patient focused and to adopt the precautionary prin-ciple – better to be safe than sorry. These apparently perfectly reasonable starting points may seem much less so when applied to a very poor household, where seeking costly treatment that is possibly not strictly necessary or of only limited benefit for one family member may entail substantial reductions in consumption expenditure for others. We would also need to consider the possibility that similar exercises could be undertaken by less scrupulous enterprises, building on the trust established by their well-intentioned competitors. The recent controversy around the future of microfinance enterprises may be relevant in this context (e.g. Aitken, 2010).

One underlying assumption of much of the debate around the new health knowledge economy is that people are moving from being essentially passive recipients of care to active participants in their treatment. One key driver of this change has been an explosive growth in the volume of health-related information flows. Many who would previously have relied on the judgements of local health providers, possibly supplemented by advice from family and friends, vaguely remembered newspaper articles or stories broadcast by local radio or television stations, now have access to, and in some case are directly targeted by, a vast array of competing sources of information. Over the past twenty years an explosive growth in the number of radio and television channels, print publications and mobile telephony- and internet-based services has resulted in a step change in the range of material available and the speed with which access is possible. Healthcare providers who have previously found it relatively easy to dismiss the doubts of those self-diagnosing from a medical dictionary or self-treatment guide are now confronted by patients who may have instant access to thousands of apparently authoritative information sources that appear to address their specific health concerns.

This revolution has been associated with the emergence of a great variety of content providers with very different aims and incentives. In addition to a diverse range of qualified and unqualified health workers, these include public health information agencies, producers and sellers of health-related goods and services, advertising and public relations agencies, international and national NGOs, advocacy groups and media companies seeking audiences. Some of these will offer valuable information and guidance. Others may dissuade seriously ill individuals from seeking appropriate treatment or encourage the worst fears of the worried well in order to sell them a guaranteed cure. The overwhelming majority will be subject to no external quality control procedures and have almost complete freedom to claim qualifications they do not possess, make wildly exaggerated or simply false statements as to the efficacy of treatments they recommend, invent evidence to support such statements and even conceal their true identities or allegiances.

This rapidly changing health knowledge economy provides both opportunities and challenges. As indicated above, one widely accepted distinguishing characteristic of health markets is the imbalance of power between possessors of expertise and those hoping to benefit from it – the problem of information asymmetry. The new technologies can in principle redress this balance. A poor woman in a Bangladesh village can use a mobile telephone to access the GrameenPhone Healthline (GrameenPhone, 2006) and ask a qualified doctor whether the drugs being prescribed by a local provider will make her condition better or worse and whether the proposed fee is reasonable. A member of an internet-based AIDS patient group can compare experiences with thousands of sympathetic fellow sufferers, some with professional expertise, and gain the confidence required to challenge sub-standard treatment. On the other hand, the capacity to communicate information faster, more often, in more attractive formats and in a much more targeted fashion offers enormous opportunities for those who wish to exploit the technologies for maximum commercial or political advantage, irrespective of the cost to specific individuals or the population at large. Medical 'quacks, charlatans, mountebanks, cranks and hucksters' (Wahlberg, 2007) have been an integral part of the history of health care, probably since its inception. They have often proved both highly adaptable to changed environments and highly innovative in their use of new technologies. It is not surprising that they have enthusiastically grasped the opportunities offered by developments in ICT.

The new technologies thus raise complex challenges in terms of equity of access to health information, the quality of that information and the trust which users can place in information providers. Mechanisms are needed that can both promote beneficial applications, for example improving the ability for service users to make better-informed choices, and limit the opportunities for misuse. They imply a need for new ways of thinking, both about the nature of regulation and about the extended range of actors and modes of accessing health information and services to which that regulation should be applied. In the OECD countries this new thinking will probably involve further development of existing institutional arrangements such as professional codes of conduct and formal regulatory regimes, which evolved partly to mediate the relationship between providers and users of expertise to mitigate the potential adverse consequences of information asymmetry. However, these are weakly developed in many developing and middle-income countries, where the combination of increasing marketization and largely unmediated access to information and services has created opportunities for harmful behaviour as well as potential gains. To highlight one obvious example, health workers, drug sellers and pharmaceuticals suppliers often have powerful incentives to encourage a costly style of medical care involving over-medicalization of self-limiting conditions and unnecessary health expenditure. Combining those incentives with a capacity to conduct extensive media-based advertising campaigns alongside highly targeted information flows to specific provider and patient groups, or even specific individuals using computer databases, the internet and mobile phones, could greatly exacerbate an already extremely worrying situation.

On the other hand, the spread of relatively low-cost information and communication technologies may also contribute to addressing such issues by providing alternative forms of knowledge mediation that can be linked to effective regulatory mechanisms. For example, the drug tracking initiatives discussed earlier in the chapter could in principle be used to address one of the most important and long-standing issues in many less-developed countries: the widespread distribution of ineffective and sometimes dangerous counterfeit drugs. ICT has the potential to disseminate expert knowledge and respond to requests for specific kinds of information, for instance through internet-linked mobile telephony, at a cost that is at least within reach of poorer populations. It can enhance the agency of local health service user groups, empowering them to create their own knowledge base and take more informed decisions, perhaps in collaboration with supportive health professionals from outside their own region. Such innovations can be locally managed, small-scale and relatively inexpensive.

Macro-level institutional arrangements in health and other social sectors are also emerging which allow the use of information technology to monitor provider behaviour and make information on that behaviour public. An interesting example is provided by recent developments in China, where the introduction of Basic Medical Insurance schemes in urban areas (Tang and Meng, 2004) and the parallel New Cooperative Medical Schemes (Mao, 2006) in rural ones has resulted in a computerized inpatient record system which, though primarily intended for accounting purposes, has considerable potential in terms of allowing local government to oversee the activities of both notionally public-sector but largely autonomous and market-oriented hospitals and private primary care providers.

The new health knowledge economy reflects the increasing role of non-state actors in health systems, particularly where markets are playing an increasing part, and raises complex governance issues. Health systems analysts often speak of public–private partnerships, but this language is inadequate to describe many of the institutional arrangements emerging at the interface between states, markets and civil society. Whether these arrangements will be adequate to guide the astonishingly complex, dynamic expansion of ICT applications in the health sector has yet to be determined.

Notes

1 www.bridges.org/publications/11/exec_summary
2 www.SIMpill.com
3 www.cell-life.org

4   www.edc.org/GLG/gkd/Sep_2001/0032.html
5   http://mobileactive.org/motech-new-approach-health-care
6   www.kiwanja.net/database/project/Project_Voxiva_Tamil.pdf
7   www.healthunbound.org/content/nacer-0
8   www.clintonglobalinitiative.org/commitments/commitments_search.asp?Section=
    Commitments&PageTitle=Browse%20and%20Search%20Commitments
9   www.mdhil.com/aboutus
10 www.poptech.org/project_m
11 www.praekeltfoundation.org/txtalert.html
12 Open-source software is freely available in a format that allows adaptation to new
    purposes and contexts.
13 www.comminit.com/en/node/310875/3076
14 www.cell-life.org/research/136-using-smss-to-reduce-loss-to-follow-up-in-pmtct
15 www.kiwanja.net
16 Open-source software provides access to the source code of applications such that third
    parties can modify it to meet their specific requirements.
17 Mobile phones that can run application software.
18 Basic mobile phones can be purchased for $15–$20 in many countries.
19 Global System for Mobile Communications.
20 Generally described as GPRS (2.5G) and EDGE (2.75G) networks.
21 These are often written in the Java programming language. Mobiles that can run
    applications written in Java are described as 'Java-enabled'. They are also often
    described as 'feature phones'.
22 Datadyne is led by Joel Selanikio, interestingly an advocate of simple SMS applications
    (www.datadyne.org).
23 For example, the Apple iPhone and Google Android devices.
24 www.androlib.com/android.application-category.list.health-Bi.aspx; www.uspharmd.
    com/blog/2009/100-fabulous-iphone-apps-for-your-health-and-fitness; www.guardian.
    co.uk/technology/2010/aug/30/iphone-replace-stethoscope
25 http://bigthink.com/ideas/20634
26 www.qualcomm.com/products_services/mobile_content_services/health
27 www.sagoodnews.co.za/science_technology/afridoctor_wins_nokia_application_
    contest.html
28 http://news.bbc.co.uk/1/hi/technology/10407081.stm
29 www.myglucohealth.net
30 http://blumcenter.berkeley.edu/global-poverty-initiatives/mobile-phones-rural-
    health/remote-disease-diagnosis
31 http://innovate.ee.ucla.edu/welcome.html
32 www.wired.com/epicenter/2010/04/sms-fights-malaria-scourge-in-africa/?utm_ source
    =feedburner&utm_medium=feed&utm_campaign=Feed%3A+wired%2Findex+%28
    Wired%3A+Index+3+%28Top+Stories+2%29%29&utm_content=Yahoo%21+Mail#i
    xzz0nkL1teHo (accessed 10 August 2010)
33 http://sproxil.com
34 www.intel.com/capital
35 www.mpedigree.net/mpedigree/index.php
36 www.securingpharma.com/40/articles/492.php
37 www.securingpharma.com/40/articles/723.php
38 http://firstcarehealth.in/servicedeliverymodel.asp
39 www.drishtee.com
40 www.sehatfirst.com/#/objectives/4527966722
41 www.robertsontechnologies.net
42 www.docs.org
43 www.unescap.org/icstd/applications/cec

44 www.grameencommunications.com/index.php/Current-Projects/village-computer-and-internet-program-vcip/
45 http://news.oneindia.in/2006/07/28/microsofts-project-saksham-for-empowering-rural-community-1154144348.html
46 Any intervention will almost always have a specified or (much more commonly) unspecified probability of success and may also involve a risk of adverse outcomes.

References

Aitken, R. (2010) 'Ambiguous incorporations: microfinance and global governmentality', *Global Networks*, 10 (2): 223–243

Amexo, M., Tolhurst, R., Barnish, G. and Bates, I. (2004) 'Malaria misdiagnosis: effects on the poor and vulnerable', *Lancet*, 364 (9448): 1896–1898

Barrington, J., Wereko-Brobby, O., Ward, P., Mwafongo, W. and Kungulwe, S. (2010) 'SMS for Life: a pilot project to improve anti-malarial drug supply management in rural Tanzania using standard technology', *Malaria Journal,* 9 (298). Online, available at: www.malariajournal.com/content/pdf/1475-2875-9-298.pdf

Blaya, J. A., Fraser, H. S. F. and Holt, B. (2010) 'E-Health technologies show promise in developing countries', *Health Affairs*, 29 (2): 244–251

Bloom, G., Standing, H. and Lloyd, R. (2008) 'Markets, information asymmetry and health care: towards new social contracts', *Social Science and Medicine*, 66 (10): 2076–2087

Boakye, K., Scott, N. and Smyth, C. (2010) *Mobiles for Development*, UNICEF, New York. Online, available at: www.cto.int/Portals/0/docs/research/mobiles4dev/UNICEF Mobiles4Dev Report for Dessemination.pdf

Breslauer, D. N., Maamari, R. N., Switz, N. A., Lam, W. A. and Fletcher, D. A. (2009) 'Mobile phone based clinical microscopy for global health applications', *PLoS ONE*, 4 (7): e6320

Chetley, A. (ed.) (2006) *Improving Health, Connecting People: The Role of ICTs in the Health Sector of Developing Countries: A Framework Paper*, Infodev, World Bank, Washington, DC

Coronado, E., Krettecos, C. and Lu, Y. (2007) 'What works: Mi Farmacita Nacional', *What Works Case Study*, World Resources Institute, Washington, DC

Drishtee Foundation (2010) Online, available at: www.drishteefoundation.org/completed_projects.html

Feder, J. L. (2010) 'Cell-phone medicine brings care to patients in developing nations', *Health Affairs*, 29 (2): 259–263

Fillip, B. and Foote, D. (2007) *Making the Connection: Scaling Telecentres for Development,* Information Technology Applications Center (ITAC), Academy for Education Development, Washington, DC

GrameenPhone (2006) Press release: 'GrameenPhone launches health information & service'. Online, available at: www.grameenphone.com/about-us/media-center/press-release/2006/176/grameenphone-launches-health-information-service (accessed 20 April 2010)

Halford, S., Lotherington, A. T., Obstfelder, A. and Dyb, K. (2010) 'Getting the whole picture', *Information, Communication and Society*, 13 (3): 442–465

Hanlon, G., Strangleman, T., Goode, J., Luff, D., O'Cathain, A. and Greatbatch, D. (2005) 'Knowledge, technology and nursing: the case of NHS Direct', *Human Relations*, 58 (2): 147–171

Hersh, W. R., Hickam, D. H., Severance, S. M., Dana, T. L., Krages, K. P. and Helfand, M.

(2006) 'Diagnosis, access and outcomes: update of a systematic review of telemedicine services', *Journal of Telemedicine and Telecare*, 12 (2): 3–31

IRIN PlusNews (2008) 'Uganda: using mobile phones to fight HIV'. Online, available at: www.plusnews.org/Report.aspx?ReportId=80176 (accessed July 2010)

Kahn, J. G., Yang, J. S. and Kahn, J. S. (2010) '"Mobile" health needs and opportunities in developing countries', *Health Affairs*, 29 (2): 252–258

Kaplan, W. A. (2006) 'Can the ubiquitous power of mobile phones be used to improve health outcomes in developing countries?', *Globalization and Health*, 2006 (2): 9.

Khan, T. (2004) *Mobile Phones Keep Track of HIV Treatments*, Science and Development Network (SciDev.Net). Online, available at: http://www.scidev.net/en/news/mobile-phones-keep-track-of-hiv-treatments.html (accessed 20 April 2012)

Mao, Z. (2006) *Pilot Program of China's New Cooperative Medical Scheme System Design and Progress*, United Nations for Economic and Social Commission for Asian and the Pacific (UNESCAP), Bangkok. Online, available at: www.unescap.org/esid/hds/issues/index.asp

Mechael, P. N. (2009) 'The case for mHealth in developing countries', *Innovations*, 4 (1): 103–118

Palmer, N., Mills, A., Wadee, H., Gilson, L. and Schneider, H. (2003) 'A new face for private providers in developing countries: what implication for public health?', *Bulletin of the World Health Organization*, 81 (4): 292–297

Paul, J. (2004) 'What works: n-Logue's rural connectivity model', *What Works Case Study*, World Resources Institute, Washington, DC

Peters, D. H., Kohli, M., Mascarenhas, M. and Rao, K. (2006) 'Can computers improve patient care by primary health workers in India?', *International Journal for Quality in Health Care*, 18 (6): 437–445

Pollack, A. M. (2001) 'Will primary care trusts lead to US-style health care?', *British Medical Journal*, 322: 964–967

Segrè, J. and Tran, J. (2008) 'What works: Careshop Ghana', *What Works Case Study*, World Resources Institute, Washington, DC

Selanikio, J. (2010) 'The mobile revolution in health care', *Americas Quarterly*, 4 (3): 64–65

Séror, A. (2001) 'The Internet, global healthcare management systems, and sustainable development: future scenarios', *Electronic Journal on Information Systems in Developing Countries*, 5 (1): 1–18

Schuster, C. and Perez Brito, C. (2011) *Cutting Costs, Boosting Quality and Collecting Data Real-Time: Lessons From a Cell Phone-Based Beneficiary Survey to Strengthen Guatemala's Conditional Cash Transfer Program*, World Bank, Washington, DC

Singh, N. (2006) 'ICTs and India's development', Department of Economics Working Paper, University of California, Santa Cruz

Skinner, D., Rivette, U. and Bloomberg, C. (2007) 'Evaluation of use of cellphones to aid compliance with drug therapy for HIV patients', *AIDS Care*, 19: 605–607

Stewart, F. (1977) *Technology and Underdevelopment*, Macmillan, London

Tang, S. and Meng, Q. (2004) 'Introduction to the urban health system and review of reform initiatives', in G. Bloom and S. Tang (eds) *Health Care Transition in Modern China*, Ashgate, Aldershot, UK

Tseng, D., Mudanyali, O., Oztoprak, C., Isikman, S. O., Sencan, I., Yaglidere, O. and Ozcan, A. (2010) 'Lensfree microscopy on a cellphone', *Lab on a Chip*, 10: 1787–1792. Online, available at: www.rsc.org/publishing/journals/LC/article.asp?doi=c003477k

UNCTAD (2009) *Information Economy Report 2009: Trends and Outlook in Turbulent Times*, UNCTAD, New York and Geneva

United Nations (2011) *Thematic Report: The Global Campaign for the Health Millennium Goals 2011: Innovating for Every Woman, Every Child*, United Nations, New York

Wahlberg, A. (2007) 'A quackery with a difference: new medical pluralism and the problem of "dangerous practitioners" in the United Kingdom', *Social Science and Medicine*, 65: 2307–2316

WHO (2006) *eHealth Tools and Services: Needs of the Member States*, Report of the WHO Global Observatory for eHealth, World Health Organization, Geneva

WHO (2010) *eHealth Intelligence Report*, multiple issues. Online, available at: www.who.int/goe/ehir/2011/january_25_2011/en/index.html

11 The economics of social franchising for health in low- and middle-income countries

David M. Bishai and Claire Champion

This chapter discusses the economic rationale for innovative service models in private-sector healthcare delivery. 'Social franchising' and other business models of healthcare delivery secure cooperation between providers and coordinating agencies in order to improve the quality of, access to and efficiency of primary health care (PHC) in the private sector.

The chapter develops a simple economic theory of healthcare production and demand that is illustrated through application to the simple cases of independent private health providers and government-operated clinics. The economic theory highlights the need for supervisory coordination above the provider's processes of care to guard the quality of care. The theory shows how social franchising models of health care can be arranged to deliver supervision and coordination of provider quality. Theoretical predictions are compared to the experience accrued in several experiments using innovative service models to improve primary health care services.

What emerges from the theory are the following predictions:

*   There will be an undersupply of financing for coordinating agencies above the level of the provider.
*   The main promise of social franchising arrangements is their potential to bring the support of donors and or governments for the quality assurance functions that are undersupplied by laissez-faire markets.
*   The quality assurance functions of social franchises are a public good that will need ongoing finance. Quality assurance operations will not develop a stable source of demand-side market support because of the inability of patients to distinguish high-quality as against mediocre-quality clinical services.

Experience to date shows that although the private providers can sustain themselves with normal profits, the coordinating agencies seldom create enough value for providers to sustain themselves on levies and royalties – yet the coordinators do create great value for society. This financial problem is the primary obstacle to the spontaneous scaling up of social franchises. Several suggestions are forwarded to improve the financial position of the coordinators.

Introduction

The goal of this chapter is to examine the ways in which innovative service models can be used to improve the quality and accessibility of primary health care (PHC) in developing countries. In this chapter, 'primary health care' is taken to mean clinical outpatient services offered at facilities. The term 'social franchising' is used to describe a variety of contractual arrangements between networks of private providers who agree with an agency to maintain service quality standards and/or to retail subsidized drugs and medical supplies that are provided by the agency. The term 'coordinating agencies' refers to administrative bodies that are able to offer in-service training, monitoring, access to subsidized inputs, and promotion of a trademark or brand name. The strategies used by the coordinating agencies and the contractual arrangements they use are analogous to those used in the business world. Nevertheless, it is important to establish what is similar and what is different between commercial enterprises and health care. Health care is similar to commerce in that it requires cooperative behavior between several parties, each with individual goals and incentives. In business, each agent pursues financial gain. Health care is different, because financial gain is seldom the solitary goal of the provider or the coordinating agencies.

The promise of innovative service models lies in their ability to accomplish several important functions in PHC. Business-style contracting can organize small providers into units that are large enough to yield returns to scale in investments in physical capital, supply chains, and in worker training and supervision. Furthermore, under outside regulation, business models can potentially arrange for cross-subsidies to help improve access to care. In order to see the problems that business models can help to solve, this chapter will set up a simple economic theory of health care. Health care will be seen as 'a scarce input into the household's production of health'. The theory identifies the two key social interests in healthcare markets as quality and access to care by disenfranchised groups. These particular aspects of healthcare delivery are 'merit goods', meaning that society has explicit goals to achieve in ensuring quality and access by the poor.[1] A third component of the health system, which will not be considered explicitly here, is the risk-spreading or 'insurance' function that needs to be carried out in society so that the unpredictably heavy consequences of illness and injury are borne equitably. The innovative service models that will be considered here will be models of primary health care *provision*, not models of health *insurance*.

The first section of the chapter sets up the theory and reviews how quality and access may falter in a laissez-faire market for private health care. The second section applies the same theory to show the potential weaknesses of a health system that is 100 per cent government owned and operated. The third section uses the theory to yield predictions about the performance of several innovative service models of healthcare provision, and the fourth section illustrates the theory using evidence from innovative service models currently operating around the world. The concluding section discusses future ways to improve the implementation of innovative service models in PHC.

A simple system of private health care

Many policymakers in public health and healthcare systems see a link between their professional activities and the health of large groups of people. But health itself cannot simply be allocated to people. The household is the key ingredient in the health of each individual, and, collectively, household decisions are what determines the health of any population (Mokyr, 1993). Most of the benefits of better health are enjoyed by household members themselves; secondary benefits of health to employers, friends, colleagues, and beleaguered healthcare providers have lesser magnitude. Consequently, most of the incentives to improve and produce individual health fall on the household.

The economic theory of firms and production processes offers useful insights into the behavioral strategies familiar in the business world, and has been used for over thirty years to describe the behavior of patients, providers and health systems. In this theory, the household is taken to be like a firm that produces a product – health – out of inputs such as food, shelter, rest and medical care. Using mathematical notation, a production function[2] is used to summarize that there is a current technological recipe for how the inputs for a product are related to the output. A production function for the health H_i of individual i can be specified as

[1] $H_i = H(\text{Food, Shelter, } Q_j, M_j, \text{ Environment})$

where Q_j is the quality of medical inputs and M_j is the amount of medical inputs of the jth type used by this individual. Quality of care refers to technical aspects of the process of care: whether the correct diagnosis was made, correct drugs prescribed, correct counseling and follow-up provided, etc. These medical inputs may take the form of medical advice, medical procedures or drugs, and may be acquired from one or multiple locations during the course of the year. In the model, each medical input is 'quality-adjusted': weighted by its quality. It is assumed that health increases with each of these inputs but that the rate of increase gets smaller with each increment of the input.[3] As will be discussed in what follows, medical providers have better knowledge than patients about the quality of services they are providing. There is an 'asymmetry' in the possession of information about quality. Information asymmetry is what makes healthcare markets different from markets for food and shelter (Arrow, 1963).

Access as a public good

Households, like firms, decide how much health to produce by weighing the rewards from better health against the rewards from other pursuits. Let us assume that households vary in income such that 5 percent of people can be considered extremely poor. Because each household must devote its own income to health production, these extremely poor households will not be able to afford substantial inputs to health and could acquire and spread contagious disease. Contagion is an externality – a by-product of private endeavors – that motivates public interest by society in the ability of each household to acquire the inputs to health. There are other potential justifications for a social concern for the accessibility of all citizens to health care: simple altruism, a fear of terrorist acts by the downtrodden poor, or a belief that health care is a human right.

Improvement as a public good

Let us imagine what would happen in an unregulated private market for PHC. In response to households' demand for health inputs M_j and Q_j, firms will obtain profit by selling medical inputs to households. In markets for goods whose quality can be evaluated by customers, prices are generally proportional to the quality of the items. Information asymmetry would make a laissez-faire market for medical care operate differently. Let us first assume that there is a way to separately measure both the volume, M_j, and the quality, Q_j, of medical care produced. For instance, to measure M_j, one might count the numbers of visits, the numbers of tablets, the numbers of procedures. One might form rating scales for each of these types of medical care to measure Q_j. For more simplicity, let us imagine that medical providers can partially separate the decisions about how much volume and how much quality to supply. The production technology for medical care would be of the form

$$[2] \quad Q_j = Q_j(E_p, K_p M_j) \text{ and } M_j = M_j(E_p, K_p Q_j)$$

where E_p and K_p are respectively the levels of effort and capital used by the private provider. Note that this model of individual private practice does *not* include inputs of effort from any other agencies that might assist private providers in producing quality and volume of services.

The quality, Q, per service produced will increase with effort and capital but decreases with the volume of service that the provider has to produce in a workday. Medical care volume, M, also increases with effort and capital, but typically decreases with the level of quality. Medical encounters tend to improve when providers spend more time with each patient. However, time spent is not an adequate proxy for quality of services because it is possible to spend a lot of time with the patient and still not offer competent services.

Because patients can easily measure the volume of care but cannot easily measure the technical quality of care, the payment agreement between patients and providers will generally be based on fee for service, not fee for quality. Assuming the providers maximize profits, their profit function can be written as

$$[3] \quad \pi_j = P_{Mj} M_j(Y_i, P_{Mj}, Q_j) - E_p - P_k K_p$$

where P_{Mj} is the price of the jth type of medical care, and $M_j(\ )$ is a demand function for the jth type of medical care, which depends on the local household incomes, Y_i, as well as price and quality. Importantly, the dependence of demand on quality may be weak if consumers have an impaired ability to observe quality. For convenience, the model sets the price of effort,[4] P_E, equal to 1, and the price of capital is depicted as P_k.

According to the classical economic paradigm, the providers choose to supply an optimal M_j^* and Q_j^* that will maximize the profit function shown in Equation [3]. The model suggests that providers will supply medical care volume, in proportion to the quantity demanded, $M_j(Y_i, P_j, Q_j)$, at any given price. In other words, supply will meet demand. If there is a shortage of healthcare workers, the medical fees (e.g. price, P_j) will be high enough to attract further entry of workers and then price will fall as the supply grows. Price will continue to fall until it meets a natural technological floor where price is exactly equal to the cost of producing the next or 'marginal' unit of service. At this point, price equals the cost of producing one more unit of service. At equilibrium, price will also equal the benefit to patients of one more unit of service.

The theory states that the provision of health care is *perfectly efficient* at this equilibrium and matters cannot be improved without an improvement in the basic technology of health care. This scenario may be 'perfectly efficient' in a technical sense, of every unit of production having no better alternative use, but efficiency need not guarantee socially desired levels of access or intangible outputs such as quality.

Because demand for medical care is well known to increase with income (Newhouse, 1981), providers will locate themselves more densely in areas with higher income. The private market can achieve an equilibrium between demand and supply of the volume of medical services, but without regulation the equilibrium is unlikely to achieve society's desired outcome regarding the accessibility of services for the poor. Furthermore, without regulatory mechanisms or the participation of coordinating agencies above the provider to address information asymmetry about the quality of each medical care, the market equilibrium will suffer from a sub-optimal supply of quality. If the demand for M_j is unresponsive to the aspects of quality that matter most for health, profit-seeking providers will have no

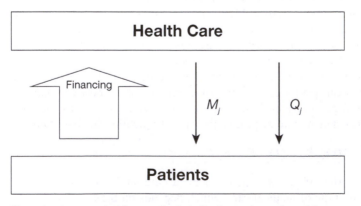

Financing is generated from patients in the form of user fees. M_j stands for the volume of medical services of type 'j'. Q_j is the quality of services of type 'j'.

Figure 11.1 Schematic diagram of a private health system.

incentive to provide quality. The medical profession addresses the medical quality problem informally by fostering professional standards among providers, by evaluating medical trainee applications for signals that the applicant is committed to putting patient welfare before private gain, and by socializing medical providers to disapprove of peers who seek to profit by under-supplying quality. Governments regulate the medical sector primarily by licensing individuals who have passed examinations and completed training in accredited institutions where they have presumably been socialized to the appropriate professional norms. Despite these mechanisms, there is abundant evidence that more could be done to improve the quality of care in the private sector of developing countries (Kumaranayake *et al.*, 2000). Saying that 'more could be done' is also saying that the model shown in Equation [2] has left out some inputs in providers' production process for service quality. Later in the chapter, we will describe in more detail the coordinating activity that could be added to the production process for service quality.

PHC in government and NGO facilities

Led by the World Health Organization and other international institutions, many countries have become substantially involved in providing PHC in hierarchical

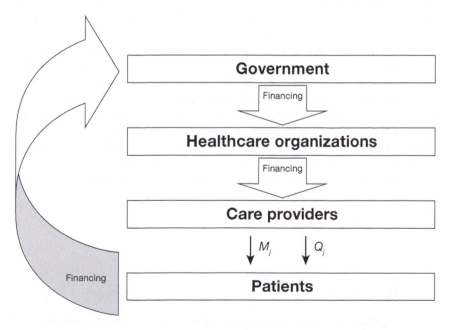

Financing is generated from patients (citizens) in the form of taxation and public borrowing. Funds are distributed to healthcare organizations, e.g. Ministry of Health, and hence to individual healthcare providers. M_j is the volume of medical services of type '*j*'. Q_j is the quality of services of type '*j*'.

Figure 11.2 Financing of a government-operated health system.

systems of community health workers, dispensaries, clinics and a tiered system of referral hospitals. In most countries the public system operates in parallel to a semi-regulated private system. Household data from several countries suggests that the majority of PHC service episodes involve private facilities (Hanson and Berman, 1998). Often the providers at the private facilities are the same individuals moonlighting after their workday at the public facilities.

Higher perceived quality in the private facilities may be one reason why households appear to prefer private-sector PHC. This may seem paradoxical in light of the last section's model of profit-seeking private providers and an undersupply of quality. However, public-sector quality may be low for reasons that parallel the problems in the private sector. Public-sector employees are paid a salary in most systems, although occasionally they may receive a 'top off' drawn from locally generated user fees. Assuming they are also profit maximizing, their profit function is of the form

[4] $\pi_G = S - E_G$

where S represents salary[5] and E_G represents the effort of government health workers multiplied by a price set equal to 1.

Since effort is costly for the public healthcare providers, they will not supply effort unless they are closely supervised or unless they derive professional satisfaction from the supply of high-quality medical care. The high degree of concern exercised in admitting and socializing applicants to the healthcare professions makes it quite possible that providers will exert themselves for the sheer satisfaction of helping other people.

The supply of government M_j and Q_j is determined by a command-and-control process heavily influenced by political forces and guesswork. The aspiration to equilibrate the supply of health services to demand is seldom realized during the process of allocating government budgets. Lacking the ability to tune the supply of services to price-borne signals of demand, governments typically under-provide capital, supplies and labor, and consequently under-produce medical services and medical quality.

[5] $Q_j = Q_j(E_G, K_G, M_j)$

and

[6] $M_j = M_j(E_G, K_G, Q_j)$

It is difficult to specify an objective function for government decision makers that is analogous to the private profit function [4]. The normative theory of the government decision maker holds that they are ideally supposed to produce the amounts of M_j and Q_j that enable each household to optimize health.[6] We lack a credible descriptive theory of what government workers actually seek to do, although some combination of achieving personal job security, getting promoted and improving public health seems plausible. It is a fact that government bureaucracies often give greater job security to those who focus on internal politics rather than the organizational mission.

Although command-and-control decision making can seldom achieve *efficient* supplies of M_j and Q_j, it can frequently surpass the private market in achieving *access* to services, and with adequate resources could surpass private market levels of *quality*. With command-and-control allocation of healthcare resources, one can deploy clinics and staff to remote or poverty-stricken areas where there are social benefits of service provision that, owing to poverty, do not result in private market demand that would attract the private sector. Indeed, by severely underpaying government workers and tacitly expecting them to moonlight (or resell government drug supplies) to make up the difference, government health ministries can apply leverage to limited budgets to achieve even more access than would be possible by paying government workers their market wage. Although the government clinics in these remote areas are shunned for their lack of drugs and quality, patients who would otherwise have no modern health provision in a remote geographical area now have a health provider, albeit one that will charge them service fees and make bootlegged drugs available for purchase. Residual problems with moonlighting providers are common to all private providers: they have weak incentives to supply high-quality care and put the patients' interests first in their treatment recommendations.

Like individual patients, elected legislators are better able to judge service volume than service quality. Elected legislative officials find it more expedient to press for more government health clinics in their home precincts than to insist that adequate salaries and quality are maintained in the current health system.

A key advantage of the government system is the potential to exploit returns to scale. The providers in the government network can potentially benefit from centrally organized training, supervision and coordination. Although the health ministries possess management plans and technical know-how that would enable them to improve quality through in-service training, the political pressure to extend access *first* has been hard to resist. In-service training and supervision do occur in government networks, but have not achieved their potential.

PHC under innovative service models for improving quality and access

In the business world there are several service industries that succeed through coordinating the activities of individual service units through an overarching administrative structure. Many NGOs have sought to emulate parts of business models in working with private healthcare providers. The franchise model has been singled out as one that is of particular interest to health care. This section will discuss the varieties of business franchising and describe the relevant issues for healthcare delivery.

Franchising: what it is

A franchise system is one where a company (the franchisor) offers a group of members (franchisees) an opportunity to sell a product or service using a business system that the franchisor developed. The core of any franchise arrangement is a contract between two specialized business partners. Franchise agreements can be used by wholesalers and retailers (as in auto dealerships), by manufacturers and wholesalers (as in soft drink bottling arrangements), or, as in the fast food industry, by business format originators and independent retail shops. The primary alternative to franchising is integration of the two business partners into a single firm.

The McDonald's Corporation is perhaps the most widely known franchise in the world. The corporation's success is due to a number of factors, not the least of which is its perfection of contractual systems between itself, its suppliers and thousands of independent owner-operators of its restaurants.

Box 11.1 The McDonald's story

In 1954, milkshake machine salesman Ray Kroc paid a visit to an unusual hamburger stand in San Bernardino, California, owned by brothers Dick and Mac McDonald. The brothers had become one of Kroc's biggest clients, and it did not take Kroc long to see from the long lines of customers that this restaurant had a winning business format. Within a month the McDonald brothers granted Kroc exclusive rights to sell franchises for their restaurant format. Kroc returned to Chicago, where he began to enlist owner operators who would pay the McDonald's Corporation a $950 start-up fee and 1.9 percent of annual sales. The McDonald brothers received 0.5 percent of sales as their royalty.

Kroc's genius lay in seeking to control the quality of each and every unit in the chain. He avoided the common practice at the time of signing away a whole territory in a franchise, which would then be doled out to individual operators beyond his control. He carefully screened each restaurant owner. Unlike other chains which sought to profit by requiring franchisees to buy marked up raw materials and supplies, the focus of the fledgling company was on increasing the sales at each individual restaurant. Despite superb attention to quality, and comfortable profits at each individual restaurant, for most of its first decade the McDonald's Corporation was teetering on the edge of bankruptcy. The solution came when an early CEO named Harry Sonneborn developed a McDonald's subsidiary called the Franchise Realty Corporation. The purpose of this subsidiary was to locate and lease restaurant sites from landowners who were willing to build McDonald's buildings on their property and then lease them back to the corporation in twenty-year leases. The McDonald's Corporation then charged its franchisees a markup of 40 percent over their own lease and insisted that each new franchisee sublease their restaurant from the corporation. Because of the growing popularity of its brand name, McDonald's could ask each franchisee to pay either the marked up rent or 5 percent of sales. This improved profits immediately. A few years later, Sonneborn would successfully approach the conservative financiers of Wall Street with this description of his company:

> I think you misunderstand the real nature of McDonald's . . . we are not basically in the food business. We are in the real estate business. The only reason we sell fifteen-cent hamburgers is because they are the greatest producer of revenue from which our tenants [McDonald's franchisees] can pay us our rent. There is nothing else that will produce the volume that food sales will, and all of our leases are based on a percentage of food sales. You can see the sales results of our units. That's the proof of what I'm telling you.
>
> (Love, 1995, p. 199)

The business format franchise has the capacity to transform motivated and hard-working people who know next to nothing about a particular industry into financially successful independent entrepreneurs. Without the training and business support they receive, most McDonald's restaurant owners would not be able to succeed in running an independent 'no name' hamburger stand. The healthcare industry is quite different, in that the potential franchisees are highly trained professionals who are usually quite capable of surviving on their own. Franchises in health care may not make or break a private practice, but they have the potential to add value to the healthcare operation by improving quality, maintaining it and signaling it to patients through the use of trademarks and brand names.

A model of franchising

Social franchises do not necessarily have to adhere to the strict contractual terms used by business franchises. Nevertheless, it is instructive to examine how the economic model of healthcare supply would depict the standard franchise contract. Whereas in Equation [2] the model of the supply of medical services involved Effort, Capital and Quality, let us now focus on the contribution of effort by the coordinating body, E_G, and effort by the franchisee, E_P, in producing medical services. The model closely follows that of Maness (1996):

[7] Local outlet revenue: $R = P_{Mj} M_j(Y_I, P_{Mj}, Q_j(E_G, E_P))$

where $M_j(\ )$ is demand, which depends on income, price and quality, $Q_j(\ )$ is quality, which depends on effort contributions, E_G is managerial effort by the coordinating body, and E_P is managerial effort by the franchisee.

Assume that M_j and Q_j increase with effort by each party.

[8]   Local outlet cost: $C = C(E_G, E_P)$

Assume that operational costs decrease, the more managerial effort is supplied by either party. This occurs because the managerial effort will identify leaner practices and ways to streamline the operations.

Equations [7] and [8] indicate the crux of the matter. Both the coordinating body and the franchisee are mutually linked to the revenue and costs of the enterprise. They cannot ignore each other. Franchisees need coordinating bodies to supply effort, and vice versa. The problem for each party is that the true effort of each cannot be observed. Since it cannot be observed, it is impossible to write an enforceable contract about how much effort each partner should supply. To motivate each other to supply effort, the provider and the coordinating body will share revenue. To model this with a linear contract, one can assume that the coordinating body retains a share, s, with $0 < s < 1$ of the revenue as royalty, and commands a starting franchise fee, F. Thus, the coordinating body's share of revenue is $sR + F - E_G$. In writing the contract to the franchisee, the coordinating body will choose s and F to maximize

[9] $sR(E_G, E_P) + F - E_G$

where $R(\ )$ is shorthand for the revenue function of equation [7].

The coordinating body will make its offer of s and F so that any franchisee is exactly indifferent between signing the contract and earning zero profits. The no-profit condition can be depicted as

[10] $(1 - s)R(E_G, E_P) - C(E_G, E_P) - F - E_P = 0$

The derivative of [10] with respect to E_P yields the providers' first-order condition to determine the optimal supply of effort under the contract. This is a constraint for the coordinating body in selecting optimal s and F.

[11] $(1 - s)dR/dE_P - dC/dEp - 1 = 0$

The coordinating body's own optimal supply of effort equation differentiating [9] is another constraint.

[12] $s\ dR/dE_G - 1 = 0$

In studying contracts very similar to this one, Maness (1996) notes that the coordinating body can always ensure that equation [10] is exactly true. If the provider is earning positive profits, the coordinating body will pick a larger franchise fee, F, or a larger royalty, s, to make the constraint bind – even though s and F may not be profit-maximizing for the provider.

A model of vertical integration

In an integrated model the linked coordinating body and franchisee solve their mutual need to elicit effort from each other by having the coordinating body retain a larger portion of revenue, sR, but pay an annual bonus, W, to the provider. Now the coordinating body chooses s and W to maximize

[13] $sR(E_G, E_P) - C(E_G, E_P) - W - E_G$

subject to the no-profit condition for the provider

[14] $(1-s)R(E_G, E_P) + W - E_p = 0$

and the optimal provider effort condition

[15] $(1-s)dR/dE_p - 1 = 0$

and the optimal coordinator's effort condition

[16] $s\, dR/dE_G - dC/dE_G - 1 = 0$

Neither party receives the full return to effort or to capital investment because of the bonus payment.

Neither the franchised contract nor the integrated contract is fully optimal because neither contract leads both parties to suffer the full penalty from withholding effort. The tendency to withhold effort is greatest for the one getting the lower share of revenue. In integrated models the provider would be more likely to

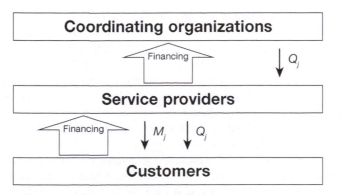

Financing for the providers is generated from customers in the form of user fees. Financing for the coordinating organization is drawn from fees and royalties paid by the service providers. M_j is the volume of services of type 'j'. Q_j is the quality of services of type 'j'

Figure 11.3 Financing of a commercially franchised system.

withhold effort. In franchised models the coordinating body would be more likely to withhold effort.

As industries choose which organizational form to use, either through rational choice or through natural selection, one would expect that integrated forms would be more common where the effort of the coordinating body is more crucial in determining revenue. Franchised forms would be more common where the effort of the individual providers is more crucial. As Maness (1996) points out, some firms never franchise (e.g. retail chains like Sears and Wal-Mart), and that would be expected if the effort by the coordinating body is more crucial in holding down costs through strategic purchases. It is quite common to see firms integrate part of their units and franchise the other part; for instance, roughly 30 percent of McDonald's restaurants are corporate-owned and corporate-operated.

Real-world experience

NGOs and charitable institutions have been operating integrated systems of private care for decades throughout the developing world. In these systems the medical providers are salaried employees of the NGO. The NGO coordinates and monitors the quality of care and is incentivized to maintain high standards of quality and access to services primarily because of professional and ideological commitments to these principles. These systems offer tremendous services to humanity, but because they rely heavily on donor support for every unit of service provided, they have limited growth potential.

Several primary health care systems have implemented 'socially' franchised systems of care. In these systems the providers support themselves through user fees, but they receive training, supplies, coordination, and use of a heavily promoted brand name from a coordinating body. The providers pay a nominal fee to the coordinating body.

Most of the evidence to date reveals the encouraging news that the individual providers are able to maintain support for their own operations through the user fees they charge. This is not too surprising: private practices are sustainable in developing countries, and network membership should not make them less sustainable. More surprising is the evidence that the franchise membership and brand name rarely add so much value to the practices that the providers are able to transfer sufficient royalties and franchise fees to the coordinating body to sustain the whole system. The coordinating bodies do not sustain themselves without outside support, although the providers can.

While the improvements in quality and access generated in social franchises are not privately valued enough to financially sustain the whole system, one could argue that quality and access in these systems are public goods that deserve to be publicly supported.

Box 11.2 Examples of socially franchised health care

KMET

The Kisumu Medical Education Trust (KMET) is a health franchise started for the purpose of reducing maternal mortality in Kenya. The project recruits obstetricians-gynecologists, general practitioners, clinical officers, nurse midwives and community health workers, and offers them:

*   a five-day training in reproductive health;
*   a supply of government-issued contraceptives;
*   a monthly visit by a KMET staff supervisor;
*   advertising;
*   access to a revolving fund that offers $1,000 loans to providers at low interest.

The project started in 1996 and has since grown to include over 160 professional health providers and 300 community health workers. Focus groups and interviews conducted among providers and clients indicate that KMET clients can detect the improved quality of care.

Clients interviewed cited reputation for quality as the most important reason for visiting a KMET member. Providers value their membership for financial reasons but more importantly for the professional satisfaction of learning to improve their services (Montagu *et al.*, 2002).

Green Star

Green Star is a joint venture partnership between Population Services International (PSI) and Social Marketing Pakistan (SMP), a USAID spin-off. SMP has managerial autonomy. Like KMET, Green Star members who are recruited receive training, use of the heavily promoted Green Star logo, below-cost contraceptive supplies, and monthly visits by Green Star's coordinating staff.

According to PSI, its mission is to improve the health of low-income and vulnerable people through social marketing. Given this objective, PSI defines sustainability in terms of enduring health impact as opposed to financial sustainability, which focuses on fiscal issues such as cost recovery. From 1995 to 2000, Green Star grew to 11,000 providers in forty cities. Green Star generates 10 million client visits per year; the majority of its clients are from low-income groups earning less than Rs 6,000 per month. Over the same period, total Pakistan oral contraceptive sales went from 1.9 million (1994) to 4.5 million in (2000). It is quite possible that the growth of oral contraceptive sales is related to the growth of Green Star.

The NGOs are still responsible for financing the coordinating network of Green Star and paying for advertising. The providers support themselves (McBride and Ahmed, 2001).

Janani

The Janani program operates in Bihar State and was started in 1996. It includes a primary network of 8,756 rural medical providers (Titli Centres) staffed by two rural medical providers from each village. These rural providers receive three days' training at one of six regional training centers. Janani also includes a smaller network of MD and MBBS doctors staffing 'Surya' clinics. The doctors receive referrals for intrauterine devices (IUDs), sterilization and abortion from the rural providers in exchange for a commission. Each doctor receives three to five days of training at a Janani clinic near headquarters. Interviews with the providers indicate that they join the network for professional prestige. Two-thirds of rural providers report an overall increase in clients. One-third report an increase in community esteem for their practices (Montagu et al., 2002).

Future directions and summary

If one accepts that social franchises are providing a public good, one may further accept that the quality and access provided by franchised networks of private providers can and should partially offset government efforts to provide access and quality. In other words, governments could potentially redirect funds away from their own efforts to achieve access and quality in government dispensaries and reroute these funds to support the coordinating bodies (but not the direct service provision) in socially franchised systems. The advantage of doing so is that the coordinating bodies of a social franchise could have as their primary outputs quality and accessibility of service. By comparison, government clinics devote much of their resources to producing the services themselves, services which are in large part private goods. Qualified medical staff are in short supply in most systems, so this proposal would not mean that government health workers would be terminated. In practice, they would be redeployed to networked, coordinated private facilities instead of their government clinics, where they receive very little coordination, training and support. Instead of making their required appearance at the government clinic from 10:00 am to 2:00 pm then disappearing to moonlight in a private practice where quality is unmonitored, they would be put into service in networks where they would support themselves officially through user fees and at the same time receive support and training from a coordinating network. Most importantly, the coordinating network could enforce the maintenance of socially beneficial sliding scales for the user fees to avoid social inequities.

Supporting the coordinating organizations through government revenue is only one option. A more creative approach to supporting the coordinating bodies would be to allow them to exploit their returns to scale in the market for capital. An individual medical provider is too small to apply for an IMF or foundation loan. By comparison, a network of 100 providers could potentially secure capital on the world market at rates as low as 4 percent. The coordinating body could then partially mark up the price of capital and administer start-up loans to private practices in the network, for example at 10 percent. The network could even offer lower rates on capital for providers working in under-served areas. Combining the coordinating body's role in quality assurance with a role as creditor would mutually enhance both roles. The coordinating body would be firmly committed to the success of each unit to avoid default and would work hard to support the needs of its debtor providers in order to qualify for future funding from the IMF. Furthermore, the providers who owe money to the coordinating body would be very attentive to the advice and support it received. This model is sketched in Figure 11.4.

In summary, privately provided medical care is an arena where privately con-sumed commodities are transacted so patients can use these products to improve their health. These privately consumed commodities have a dual nature as public

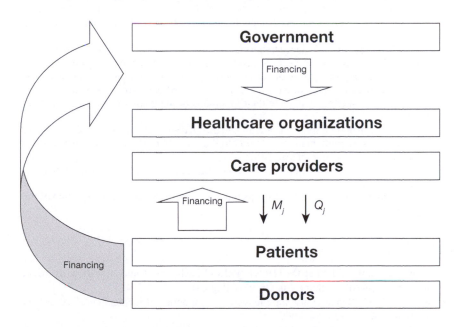

Financing for the providers is generated from patients (citizens) in the form of user fees. Financing for the healthcare organization that coordinates providers is drawn from public loans or public financing. M_j is the volume of medical services of type 'j'. Q_j is the quality of services of type 'j'.

Figure 11.4 Financing of a socially franchised system.

goods. Investment to assure the technical quality of the medical providers in a community or network is a good that can be enjoyed by all who visit those medical providers. Similarly, inasmuch as all societies have some experience with underprivileged minorities, institutional changes that improve the access to health care by the poor will be considered a public good by all who are concerned about the groups with low access. Social franchises are a potential way to finance the ongoing support needs of quality assurance personnel who might serve the private sector. They can also be used to target vulnerable populations by preferentially offering subsidized goods that appeal to the under-served minorities.

Notes

1   Not all healthcare utilization events count as merit goods. If a highly privileged person goes abroad to receive elective surgery, paid for out of pocket, this would be a relatively unimportant issue for policy. The important issues are ensuring that people are informed about the quality of services and ensuring that there are few barriers to care for the vulnerable groups in the population.
2   For instance, the production function for a peanut butter sandwich could be sketched generally as Peanut Butter Sandwich = (Peanut Butter, Jelly, Bread, Labor). This production function is shorthand for what may be a more detailed mathematical depiction of the process: 1 PB sandwich = 1 × TBSP PB + 1 × tsp Jelly + 2 × bread slices + 3 × minutes of chef time. The household can use this technological recipe to determine how much of the ingredients to acquire after first determining how many peanut butter sandwiches to produce.
3   Although the quality of food, shelter and environment matters as well, this is not depicted above. Millions of years of evolution have culled human beings who lacked skill in recognizing the quality of various offerings of food and shelter. The historical novelty of effective and potentially dangerous medical care makes it vital for individuals to somehow overcome their ignorance of the quality of medical inputs to their health.
4   Effort is more than time spent on care for patients; it also refers to the complexity of the medical decisions being made in addition to the time spent setting prices for services (American Academy of Pediatrics, 1999).
5   Actually, S is more than money – for example, the stream of benefits (job security, post-retirement benefits, etc.).
6   Readers should have little difficulty rejecting the normative theory as a depiction of the way things really are.

References

American Academy of Pediatrics (1999) 'RBRVS, what is it and how does it affect pediatrics?', AAP brochure, Elk Grove Village, IL
Arrow, K. J. (1963) 'Uncertainty and the welfare economics of medical care', *American Economic Review*, 53: 941–969
Hanson, K. and Berman, P. (1998) 'Private health care provision in developing countries', *Health Policy and Planning*, 12: 195–211
Kumaranayake, I., Lake, S., Mujinja, P., Hongoro, C. and Mpembeni R. (2000) 'How do countries regulate the health sector? Evidence from Tanzania and Zimbabwe', *Health Policy and Planning*, 15: 357–367
Love, J. F. (1995) *McDonald's: Behind the Arches*, Bantam Books, New York

McBride, J. and Ahmed. R. (2001) 'Social franchising as a strategy for expanding access to reproductive health services', Commercial Market Strategies Project, US Agency for International Development, Washington, DC

Maness, R. (1996) 'Incomplete contracts and the choice between vertical integration and franchising', *Journal of Economic Behavior and Organization*, 31: 101–115

Mokyr, J. (1993) 'Technological progress and the decline of European mortality', *American Economic Review*, 83: 324–330

Montagu, D. (2002) 'Clients of social franchises: behavior and beliefs', paper presented at the Population Association of America 2002 annual meeting, Atlanta, GA

Montagu, D., Bradbury, K. and Rogo, K. (2002) *KMET: Private Provider Network of the Kisumu Medical and Education Trust*, World Bank, Washington, DC

Newhouse, J. P. (1981). 'The demand for medical care services: a retrospect and prospect', in J. van der Gaag and M. Perlman (eds) *Health, Economics, and Health Economics*, North-Holland, New York

12 Conclusions

Making health markets work better for poor people

Gerald Bloom, Barun Kanjilal, Henry Lucas, David H. Peters and Hilary Standing

From working with private providers to engaging with health markets

As the cases presented in this book show, health stakeholders and policy analysts need to pay much more attention to the operation of the health markets that play such an important role in most low- and middle-income countries. The kinds of health systems that will eventually emerge in these countries will be strongly influenced by the degree to which governments and other stakeholders can build institutional arrangements that both encourage innovation and influence the provision of safe, effective and affordable health services.

Much of the available evidence on the performance of health markets in low- and middle-income countries comes from studies of donor-funded interventions aimed at improving the performance of private providers and/or at using public funds to purchase services from private providers. Many of these interventions were designed in the context of long-standing debates about whether 'developing countries' should adopt an 'American' or 'European' model of health system organization. These debates have strongly influenced the way the issue has been framed, generating a lot of heat about alternative visions of ideal future health systems but shedding little light on the real situation in many countries. The extraordinary economic dynamism of a number of low- and middle-income countries and the effect of the economic crisis on the United States and Europe has reduced the plausibility that either can provide a model for health system organization in the rest of the world (Crisp, 2010).

The chapters in this book show that health markets have become a very important source of drugs and outpatient medical care for poor people and that the development of appropriate institutional arrangements to influence the performance of these markets has lagged behind their growth. In consequence, poor and vulnerable people are at risk of receiving dangerous and/or ineffective medical care and spending unnecessarily large amounts of money on these services. They also show that the dichotomous definition of health service providers as either 'public' or 'private' bears little resemblance to reality. In China, for example, formal ownership by a local government is only one of a number of influences on the performance of facilities that rely on market activities for financial survival.

In Bangladesh and India the boundary between what is public and what is private is obscured by the movement of health workers into market-based practice simultaneously with their formal service, and complex referral linkages across the boundary. In Cambodia a national NGO has emerged to help poor people with diabetes negotiate medical support in managing their illness in the context of unregulated health markets and a government system that can only meet a small proportion of the potential demand for services. These case studies illustrate the need to move beyond a narrow focus on the formal ownership of providers of health-related goods and services and to build a greater understanding of the complex health market systems that now exist in many countries. The remainder of this chapter outlines elements of a strategy for supporting the creation of appropriate institutional arrangements for increasing access to effective and affordable health services in contexts of rapidly changing market economies.

Building knowledge of health market systems

The first step towards more effective engagement with health markets is to create a body of systematic knowledge on their structure and the factors that influence their performance. The health market systems approach outlined in Chapter 1 provides a framework for analysing influences on the performance of providers of health-related goods and services. These include:

- formal ownership of organizations and their mission;
- the relationship between organizations that finance and provide health services and the pattern of incentives the providers face;
- government bodies (national and local) with mandates to influence different aspects of the performance of health organizations;
- professional and business associations, citizen groups, mechanisms of local accountability and other civil society organizations that influence health systems;
- formal and informal norms of behaviour that are widely accepted as part of a social contract in the health sector;
- political factors and the basic elements of regime legitimacy.

The findings of a health market systems analysis can be used in the design and implementation of interventions to improve the performance of these markets in meeting socially agreed objectives. The case studies illustrate a variety of interventions that involve government, market arrangements (such as different forms of franchising) and existing or new civil society organizations. They demonstrate the complexity of these interventions and the need for all relevant stakeholders to learn new roles and responsibilities in ensuring that health markets take into account the needs of the general public, as well as the interests of specific stakeholders.

Understanding sources of innovation

There are a number of sources of innovations with the potential to improve substantially the performance of health markets in low- and middle-income countries. The advanced market economies have spawned a number of market-driven organizational models that include retail pharmacy and hospital chains, and franchises for a variety of health-related products. These models are diffusing through the expansion of organizations to other countries and by replication of these models by local entrepreneurs. Several donor programmes have attempted to adapt these models to meet the needs of the poor, but there is little evidence, to date, about the degree to which these efforts have successfully altered the performance of a health market system.

The rapid economic growth of a number of low- and middle-income countries is creating new international centres for technological and organizational innovation (Mashelkar, 2005; Leadbeater and Wilsdon, 2007). The demand for health-related goods and services is rising very rapidly in these countries. This increased demand is likely to result in the emergence of quite different types of market organization that reflect current technologies, the economic and social context, and the regulatory environment in these countries. If these companies can build a reputation for providing trustworthy services at an affordable price, they could expand very rapidly to become important actors in the global health economy. This process is well advanced in the pharmaceutical sector and there are already signs of the emergence of large service delivery companies. The rapid development of information and communications technology is creating major opportunities for new kinds of organization, such as mobile phone health companies, to play a potentially disruptive role in the organization of the health sector.

The emergence of pluralistic health systems attests to the volume of local innovation. One commonly finds a bewildering variety of providers of health-related goods and services in many different practice settings. One can also find many examples of local approaches to build trust and address information asymmetry. The major lack has been in mechanisms to associate these providers with larger-scale organizations to extend access to the benefits of healthcare technology to larger segments of the population.

There is growing interest in the role of social entrepreneurs in health-related markets. The term is usually used to refer to organizations that 'borrow a mix of business, charity and social movement models to reconfigure solutions to community problems and deliver sustainable new social value' (Nicholls, 2006, p. 2) and/or to a focus on the creation of social value and a number of attributes of innovation, risk taking and a willingness to try something new (Peredo and McLean, 2006; Weerawardena and Mort, 2006). Social entrepreneurs work in the public, private and social sectors and are often involved in organizational innovations across these sectors. This makes them particularly interesting in the context of heavily marketized health systems with blurred boundaries between public and private roles and functions.

The boundary between social entrepreneurship and responses to commercial opportunities can shift. For example, banking through mobile telephones has evolved from being an act of social entrepreneurship to a major business opportunity. The same applies to micro-credit. An assessment of micro-credit confirms its success in achieving growth in access by people previously excluded from the organized economy (Greeley, 2006). It has substantially improved the performance of credit markets by using innovative approaches for identifying good credit risks, appropriate to the institutional context of many low-income countries. Successful schemes are linking to commercial financial organizations. This in turn may create new ways of delivering insurance-based health protection.

There is a significant risk that organizational innovations will create new types of market segmentation in which more people are able to benefit from efficient markets, but some are still excluded. In this context, Greeley (2006) points out that there is limited evidence that the very poorest people have benefited from commercial micro-credit. He emphasizes the importance of monitoring the performance of innovations in meeting the needs of the poor. Measures to meet the needs of the excluded are almost certainly going to require subsidies from government or other sources, with associated specialized institutions to ensure that these subsidies reach the target population.

Strengthening health market systems

In this section we draw on the analysis of health market systems and the case studies to present an initial framework for making health-related markets work better in meeting the needs of the poor. What this book has drawn attention to is the need to go well beyond the immediate context of local suppliers and users – the interactions between 'private' providers and users of goods and services in health systems. These interactions are part of complex health market systems that vary in many particulars and are embedded in contextually specific social, political and economic environments and associated institutional arrangements, spanning the local to the global. Whereas there is much to be learned and adapted across different contexts, 'what works' will be a balance between more generic findings and innovations that draw from specific experience. We have argued that institutional innovation will arise predominantly from this intersection.

Table 12.1 provides a descriptive matrix that brings together the major components influencing health market systems. Innovations aimed at changing provider performance are unlikely to result in sustainable changes to health market systems unless complemented by changes to other aspects of the market system. Such changes may involve the creation and enforcement of new regulations, the engagement of a variety of actors in regulatory and/or accountability partnerships and the development of new mechanisms of accountability in strengthening access to reliable and trustworthy knowledge. It is impossible to separate the performance of the supplier organizations from the market system within which they are embedded. Thus, in assessing the challenges and viability of an intervention or innovation a key step is to map it in relation to the wider health market system.

Table 12.1 Health market systems framework for mapping of interventions

Market factors	Supporting functions and rules	Product variation	Product organizational attributes	Institutional factors	Market and non-market actors engaged in producing market order
Level of formalization	Infrastructure	Level of: Clinical/ practitioner skill	Managerial competence	Payment systems, both by patients and to practitioners	Formal regulatory authorities – local, national, international
Degree of information asymmetry	Information flows	Clinical/ practitioner effort	Financial resources – quantity	Segregation or integration of various medical services	Informal organizations, local, national, international
Degree of segmentation	Related services	Clinical/ practitioner integrity (trustworthiness)	Financial resources – source		
	Laws				
Complexity of supply chain	Sector-specific regulations and standards	Price	Governance structure (and its alignment with patient interests) – ownership; values; extent of patron-clientage; influence of financial source	Extent and quality of external state regulation of quality	'Hybrids', e.g. private or independent agencies with 'public' mandate
Interconnectedness of markets	Informal rules and norms including those of health workers	Accessibility – subdivided into distance, hours of practice, languages spoken and social distance		Extent and quality of external and internal regulation of quality by professions and other associations	Private companies
Global, national and local market systems	Non-statutory regulations/codes				NGOs/non-state service provider organizations
Source/driver(s) of innovation	Social values	Level of: Patient knowledge		Extent of implicit regulation and training	Providers' associations

Patient effort (including compliance)
Patient trust (note that a patient may trust a provider who is not trustworthy)
Patient ability to pay

provided by the referral system

Extent and quality of internal regulation of quality by the health organization

Visibility of reputation, including via franchises, 'report cards', and sharing of experience between neighbours

Interrelationship with global organizations and institutions

Citizens' bodies, co-producing arrangements

User organizations

Media and other sources of health-related information

This mapping process provides a basic template for situating an intervention or innovation in relation to market functions, players and potential institutional arrangements. It provides the basis for a series of further questions to be asked about the potential to achieve the following outcomes:

- Does it reduce information asymmetry and enable patients to better assess whether the health services they are acquiring are appropriate to their condition?
- Does it align incentives better or worse with patient welfare?
- Does it relieve or exacerbate constraints on competence, finance and management?
- Is there evidence that it results in better health-related outcomes?
- Does it provide benefits to the poor and does it support the creation of sustainable arrangements to meet the needs of the poor in the longer term?
- Is it likely to encourage innovation and support the development of a more coherent market, or is it likely to distort the market and be purely temporary?

The devil, then, is in the detail. The evolution of market actors depends strongly on the specific interactions between direct financial incentives and the countervailing influences of reputation and a variety of regulatory and accountability arrangements. Successful management of institutional change involves the construction of new rules and widely shared understandings of what constitutes legitimate and illegitimate behaviour. A paper on the factors that influence the investment climate in developing countries by Moore and Schmitz (2008) contrasts an idealized view that advocates the construction of highly organized institutional arrangements as a prerequisite to economic growth with a messier reality within which private actors create informal arrangements to facilitate trust-based market transactions, and governments establish mutually beneficial relationships with private actors to create some degree of market order. Moore and Schmitz argue that the political economy strongly influences the degree to which these arrangements lead to economic growth and the eventual creation of rules-based market order, or to a descent into low-efficiency 'crony capitalism'.

Similar factors influence the trajectory of health-related markets in which informal arrangements and a variety of partnerships between governments and private actors play important roles. In some circumstances the state is unlikely to do more than prevent very dangerous practices such as the sale of counterfeit drugs, leaving local actors to create informal arrangements to bring some order to health-related markets. These arrangements are unlikely to be efficient except with regard to very simple goods and services. In other circumstances the state and/or other actors play a leadership role in a process that can eventually lead to a rules-based regulatory system. Where state regulatory capacities are weak, it may be possible to create alternative institutions that can improve quality, but not in a manner that is economic in the short run. These changes are likely to demand philanthropic or donor investments that will see the new institution through the period in which it is gaining recognition in the market of health consumers.

Countries face a major challenge in managing a transition from a situation of largely chaotic and inefficient health-related markets to more ordered market systems underpinned by some form of social contract. This transition will involve experimentation and learning by a number of actors and the gradual development of appropriate rules, behavioural norms and mutual expectations. The Chinese use a compelling metaphor to describe their management of multiple transitions as 'crossing the river while feeling for the stones'. This captures the iterative nature of a process that is driven by local innovation and adaptation and where a legal and regulatory framework is evolving to incorporate lessons from local innovations that have worked well or have been developed as responses to scandals or major negative outcomes. It is much too early to assess the success of China's efforts to improve the performance of its health system, and there is lots of room for debate about the applicability of this approach to countries with very different administrative and political systems. Nonetheless, this metaphor encapsulates an important message about the kind of complex change process that many countries will need to manage in their health-related markets. This change process will involve a number of stakeholders learning new roles and responsibilities to ensure that services are safe and effective and that they meet the needs of the entire population, including the poor. It needs to be accompanied by the creation of new rules of behaviour underpinned by ethical norms. The kinds of institutions that emerge from this process will strongly influence the pathways of health system development for many years to come.

Final thoughts: a framework for learning and dissemination of lessons

It should be clear from the diverse examples provided in this volume that there are no simple blueprints for the creation of both appropriate health service delivery organizations and the institutional arrangements to influence their performance in meeting the needs of the poor. The lack of simple blueprints highlights the importance of a learning approach that enables relevant actors to learn how local health markets work and to test alternative institutional innovations. As an initial step, building on work on learning approaches in development (Brinkerhoff and Ingle, 1989; Bond and Hulme, 1999), we propose a conceptual framework that recognizes key market players and institutions and focuses on the concrete activities they can undertake (Figure 12.1). This framework is not only a reflection of how public institutions may have been designed (e.g. with assumptions about Weberian motivations), or how they currently operate, for instance as dependent on street-level bureaucrats or front-line staff who use their discretion in implementing central policies (Lipsky, 1980). Nor is it limited to learning processes within private or civil society organizations. Rather, this is an action-oriented framework that builds on all these experiences.

The framework shown in Figure 12.1 is intended to be a flexible guide to different types of learning process, and its application is expected to vary considerably depending on local market conditions. At different stages in the design and

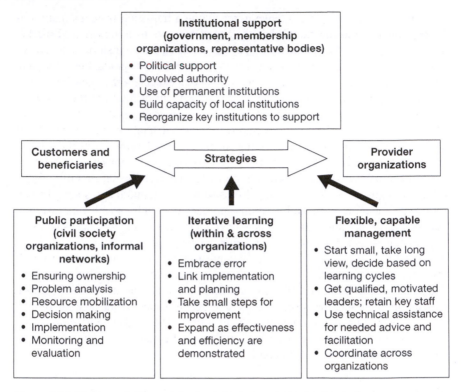

Figure 12.1 Framework for applying systematic learning to health markets.

implementation of strategies to improve the provision of health-related goods and services, a variety of actors will play important roles. For example, consumer organizations may be directly involved in problem solving, resource mobilization and monitoring. Yet consumer organizations do not necessarily represent the interests of the poor (Peters and Muraleedharan, 2008), which may lead to continued negotiations of formal and informal rules between their stakeholders and the organization. The interests of consumer organizations may also be in conflict with those of providers or other key players, which may result in providers being less forthcoming with information, or less willing to collaborate. Service provider organizations will work best if they are able to identify and retain qualified and motivated staff, communicate effectively across organizations, and use professional facilitation and advice in targeted ways (as distinct from the tendency in many development agencies to see technical assistance as a driving force for change). Critical institutional support includes government policies that encourage local participation and innovation by service providers, using permanent and local organizations for administration and regulatory functions, and a willingness and ability to reorganize and refocus these institutions as needs are identified.

A common problem in the health sector in developing countries is limited capacity for implementation of strategies. Trying to find the right fit between intervention goals, the expectations of beneficiaries or customers, and the capabilities of implementing organizations, governments and communities is an ongoing challenge. We propose that part of the solution involves continually questioning capacity constraints and being aware of the effects on other market players. Do the constraints lie in the lack of specific human skills, infrastructure or management systems that organizations need to perform their work, or is there a more important problem in the setting and enforcing of rules across organizations, or in communicating information between different actors? If the constraints lie within a key organization, such as a service provider or regulatory agency, radical reorganization is often considered, even though the costs to morale and productivity can be substantial. Can such problems be addressed by more subtle changes that minimize these costs while better aligning responsibilities, authorities, resources and accountabilities with the objectives and tasks of the organization?

Knowing when the pace of change is outstripping the ability of organizations to deliver quality services effectively requires intelligence gathering and processing with both implementers and service beneficiaries. Simply asking which units within an organization appear to be performing well and which do not may provide early warning signs. Although any well-functioning organization will try to monitor the performance of its own constituent units, government regulatory agencies are traditionally seen as having the main role in assessing performance across organizations. In health market systems, however, the leading players in assessment, and in setting rules on provider performance, may also include consumer groups, research agencies, the media, professional bodies or insurance companies. Whatever the origin of information concerning provider performance, it is important to consider the roles of other market players and their responses to that information.

Processes that encourage learning and good decision making

A range of existing tools can be applied to reinforce iterative learning that links implementation and planning, encourages appropriate risk taking and promotes a forward-thinking perspective towards expansion of services that builds on what is learned. Participation in learning processes across organizations involves risks, as it cannot be assumed that stakeholders will always see a benefit in their participation. A culture within organizations that accepts error may be needed, as well as trust between organizations. In the absence of trust, actors may undermine learning processes by manipulating information.

Processes that encourage learning, decision making and action based on learning have been shown to be particularly effective in improving implementation (Peters *et al.*, 2009). There is little evidence to suggest that specific types of organization must take a lead in driving or facilitating such processes in a given context. They tend to rely on the involvement of multiple stakeholders.

Types of question to ask in a learning strategy

On the basis of an extensive review of strategies that have been used to improve the performance of health workers and health service organizations, a number of key questions and strategies have been identified as associated with good learning strategies. These include the following:

*   Are there positive and negative outliers in providing health services? For example, are there differences between states within a country, communities within a district, or neighbourhoods within a community? Are there differences between vulnerable groups and other segments of society? Are there differences across different service delivery organizations? Differences may exist in terms of high and low performance or in population groups. Look for a range of available sources of data, including both routine health information systems and informal mechanisms, for example key informants or the media. Consider the way in which analysis is related to actions taken by decision-makers, be they front-line providers of services, managers within a service delivery organization, senior executives or policy-makers, or regulatory and membership bodies.
*   What are the unintended consequences of the strategy? When implementing health interventions, most people tend to look only at the intended results, but it is also important to look at any possible unintended consequences outside the narrow focus of the intervention itself.
*   Does the strategy create the right incentives for critical organizations and people to work towards a common purpose? Changes in laws, regulations, leadership, macro organization changes, or economic or political shocks can radically affect the way health services are implemented. Trying to anticipate many of these shocks may be very difficult, but it may be more important to be able to recognize when they are occurring as soon as possible, and to take corrective steps. This again involves good information gathering and feedback mechanisms.

One conclusion of the proposed learning-based approach is that interventions and institutional changes should not be undertaken in isolation. One reason is to be able to identify and address the unintended consequences of any reform effort or attempt to influence markets; they are likely to affect the different players differently. Another reason is that partnerships are needed, not only to ensure sufficient scale of service provision but also to construct new social contracts and institutional arrangements within which providers are embedded. There are many learning technologies and processes that should be integral parts of any major efforts to strengthen health market systems, but it is just as important that they should involve all actors likely to influence their outcomes. If the outcomes are to benefit the poor, their participation in learning processes to influence health markets is particularly important, along with institutional arrangements that focus on achieving these benefits.

References

Bond, R. and Hulme, D. (1999) 'Process approaches to development: theory and Sri Lankan practice', *World Development*, 27 (8): 1339–1358

Brinkerhoff, D. and Ingle, M. D. (1989) 'Integrating blueprint and process: a structured flexibility approach to development management', *Public Administration and Development*, 9 (5): 487–503

Crisp, N. (2010) *Turning the World Upside Down: The Search for Global Health in the 21st Century*, Royal Society of Medicine Press, London

Greeley, M. (2006) 'Microfinance impact and the MDGs: the challenge of scaling-up', IDS Working Paper 255, Institute of Development Studies, Brighton

Leadbeater, C. and Wilsdon, J. (2007) *The Atlas of Ideas: How Asian Innovation Can Benefit Us All*, Demos, London. Online, available at: www.demos.co.uk

Lipsky, M. (1980) *Street-Level Bureaucracy; Dilemmas of the Individual in Public Services*, Russell Sage Foundation, New York

Mashelkar, R. (2005) 'Nation building through science and technology: a developing world perspective', *Innovation Strategy Today*, 1 (1): 16–32

Moore, M. and Schmitz, H. (2008) 'Idealism, realism and the investment climate in developing countries', IDS Working Paper 307, Institute of Development Studies, Brighton

Nicholls, A. (2006) 'Introduction', in A. Nicholls (ed.) *Social Entrepreneurship: New Models of Sustainable Social Change*, Oxford University Press, Oxford

Peredo, A. and McLean, M. (2006) 'Social entrepreneurship: a critical review of the concept', *Journal of World Business*, 41: 56–65

Peters, D. H. and Muraleedharan, V. R. (2008) 'Regulating India's health services: to what end? What future?' *Social Science and Medicine*, 66: 2133–2144

Peters, D. H., El Seharty, S., Siadat, B., Vujivic, M. and Janovsky, K. (eds) (2009) *Implementing Health Services Strategies in Low and Middle Income Countries: From Evidence to Learning and Doing*, World Bank, Washington, DC

Weerawardena, J. and Mort, G. (2006) 'Investigating social entrepreneurship: a multi-dimensional model', *Journal of World Business*, 41 (1): 21–35

Index